I0781807

Everything will be okay
an achondroplasia diary
by Nathalia Blair

Dedication

I dedicate this book to my daughter, all the people with achondroplasia, and the parents of children with achondroplasia.

To the children who have died because of a lack of knowledge about achondroplasia and lack of testing, this book is dedicated to your memory.

Acknowledgment

Writing this book was not easy. Writing about our daughter's health struggles was even more difficult. During this experience, I kept a journal so I would not struggle remembering dates, surgeries, or emotional experiences. Thank you God, for being with us and carrying us when we struggled, for your love and blessings, and for choosing us to be the parents of this child.

Albert Einstein said "There are only two ways to live your life. One is as though nothing is a miracle. The other is as though everything is a miracle" This book is proof that everything is a miracle. Every person who was and still in our journey is a miracle for us, are angels that God sent to us to help us, support us, push us, teach us and learn with us.

Thank you to my children because I would not be who I am today without you. My son, you taught me to be a mom and the meaning of unconditional love. My daughter, you gave me strength to fight for you. You showed me that I am stronger than I ever thought. You both taught me to overcome my fears and to be a better human. You both showed me that with love and God everything is possible. I love you both so much.

To my father, I am deeply grateful for your unconditional love and support and for always being there for us. Thank you for caring for our son while we were at the hospital and for your undying love for our children. We are so blessed.

To my mother, who fought tirelessly alongside me as I fought for my children, I can never thank you enough. You bore the brunt of my chaotic emotions yet continued to support me when I leaned on you to keep from falling. You drove me to my appointments when I was too tired and emotionally exhausted to drive myself. How many times did you wait outside for me? After spending many hours in the NICU with my child, you picked me up when I called you at three in the morning. I am in awe that you held your emotions together until your granddaughter came home. Thank you for walking every step with me.

To my siblings and in-laws, thank you for your love and support for every great and small achievement. It means so much that you were there. Thank you for your prayers. Sisters I know you are thousands of miles away but I always felt like you both were next to me.

To my husband, thank you for your support. When you discovered our daughter's possible diagnosis, you said she would be the most beautiful little person. You held my hand while we waited for our beautiful daughter to arrive and carried her soon after her birth when I could not. Thank you for loving our children and being there for our daughter. You did not treat her differently because of her diagnosis. You always saw her perfect and with love.

To my cousin Gonzalo, who prayed with me every day of my pregnancy. I would be always deeply grateful.

To my friends and new friends, thank you for your prayers, love, and support.

To my Aunts for their love and for praying and for checking on me and my daughter every single day.

To my friend Cecilia, for all your help, for letting me stay at your house with my son so I can be near to my daughter and spend time with my son, for your love, attention and friendship.

To my friend Maria Eugenia, for all your help, dedication, love and support when my daughter was struggling with her skin, your knowledge and patience were amazing.

To my Aunt Nena, for your patience and love and all your help on taking care of my two kids and for your collaboration on this book.

To our Neurosurgeon Dr. Michael Muhonen for all your support and knowledge, for answering all my concerns at any day or time and for your collaboration on this book.

We sincerely thank the doctors, nurses, home health nurses, other medical professionals, and ancillary services who supported us on this journey. Their talent, understanding, and professionalism helped us to help our daughter succeed.

We met our friends, Nathan and Rebecca Campobasso, when my husband and I raised miniature chickens, and I was pregnant with our son. They fell in love with the tiny chickens and bought some hen pets. From then on, a special friendship grew where we spoke, shared photos, and enjoyed their delicious home-cooked Italian meals. I remember Nathan speaking Italian to our daughter when he met her. "Bellissima bambina," he said. "Beautiful baby."

Rest In Peace, Nathan. We love you and miss you.
Thank you, Rebecca, for your friendship and for always being there for me. Is an honor to be your friend. Thank you for helping me research and write this beautiful story about our daughter. This book will not be possible without your help. We will be forever grateful.

Moreover, to those reading this book, I want you to know you are not alone, and everything will be okay.
Thank you God because without you nothing is possible.

Preface

According to Medical News Today, about 80% of children born with the FGFR3 gene that causes achondroplasia have average-height parents. If a child has one or both parents with this form of dwarfism, the chances are high that they, too, will inherit the FGFR3 gene.

Children who inherit two copies of the gene, one from each parent, may have severe achondroplasia. These infants typically have extreme shortening of the bone and underdeveloped rib cages and are usually stillborn or die shortly after birth from respiratory failure.

Medical care for people with achondroplasia is challenging. What needs to be improved upon is information and education that could bring awareness to the achondroplasia diagnosis, not only in infants but in their transition into adulthood.

Part One
The Parents

Achondroplasia (a-kon-dro-play-shah) (*Pereira, 2019*) is a genetic mutation. It is the most common form of disproportionate dwarfism, with 1 in 26,000 to 28,000 live births. An achondroplasia birth may have many medical complications. Knowing which medical facilities and doctors have experience handling each child's unique needs is essential.

My name is Nathalia. My husband and I have two beautiful children. Our daughter has achondroplasia, a form of dwarfism. Our world turned upside down when we found out about her diagnosis of achondroplasia. It was not her diagnosis that frightened us but the potential health complications that usually accompany it.

When reading this, I do not want you to think, "Oh, how the mother suffered and struggled with this child!" I did not suffer or struggle. More than ever, I wanted this child; I had dreamed about this child.

Some characteristics of achondroplasia can be visualized, like short arms and legs, a prominent head, and starfish hands. Some complications related to achondroplasia are not visible, like those our daughter experienced, such as brainstem compression, obstructive and central apnea, and hydrocephalus.

We do not know until after birth and sometimes during the first couple of years what problems we will encounter. I want parents to be alert for signs of common complications in these children. I do not wish to scare expectant mothers, but I do want to educate them on a plan of action for achondroplasia.

This is the story of my pregnancy, our beautiful daughter's birth, and how we learned to recognize achondroplasia complications and speak for our daughter.

Peru was my birthplace, a beautiful nation on the western

coast of South America. After I received my degree in 2003 from a college in Lima, Peru, we immigrated to California, United States. Spanish was my first language; I did not learn English until we moved to the United States.

I grew up in a close-knit Catholic family in a small city where everyone knew everyone. My parents raised four beautiful children over forty years of a happy marriage: one boy and three girls. Since my early teens, I had wished to have five children. However, that was not to be.

I married late at age thirty-two to a sweet, handsome man with sea-blue eyes. Soon after we met, our relationship moved quickly. Despite our differences in religion, culture, and language, we shared many common interests. We talked about music, books, our philosophical outlook, and how we would combine the best of both cultures and life experiences.

We had long talks about depression and anxiety; I had experienced it in the past, and he lived with chronic depression. Opening up about this early in our relationship made communicating and appreciating each other easier. Unaddressed emotional health issues can become serious when there is no one to talk to who understands you. We talked about our experiences and how we dealt with them then; we empathized with each other.

My husband shared the book Marcus Aurelius Meditations with me. The book was the diary of a Roman Emperor who suffered from depression over a thousand eight hundred years ago. Depression has a long history, but we know more about its potential causes and treatments today as it is more open to discussion.

If we were having a bad day, we would send each other a Marcus Aurelius quote to help us through whatever we were going through. We started reading and writing about Marcus Aurelius' Meditations and sharing our experiences with others.

We created a Marcus Aurelius meditation group in English and Spanish. These meditations helped us learn from and about each other, gave a deeper meaning to how our different cultures treated this once-taboo subject and helped to strengthen our relationship.

We fell in love and married in August 2015. We spent our first year and a half of marriage listening to music, reading and writing philosophy, gardening, and raising hundreds of miniature game hens in our family's large backyard.

Rearing miniature game hens and planting and growing our stunning garden of sunflowers, berries, tomatoes, and mint were fantastic therapies for depression. Our dreams were to use our game hens and gardening knowledge to help older people and others overcome or deal with depression. We felt this would be good therapy for children with depression and autism. My husband and I flourished when we took on those endeavors.

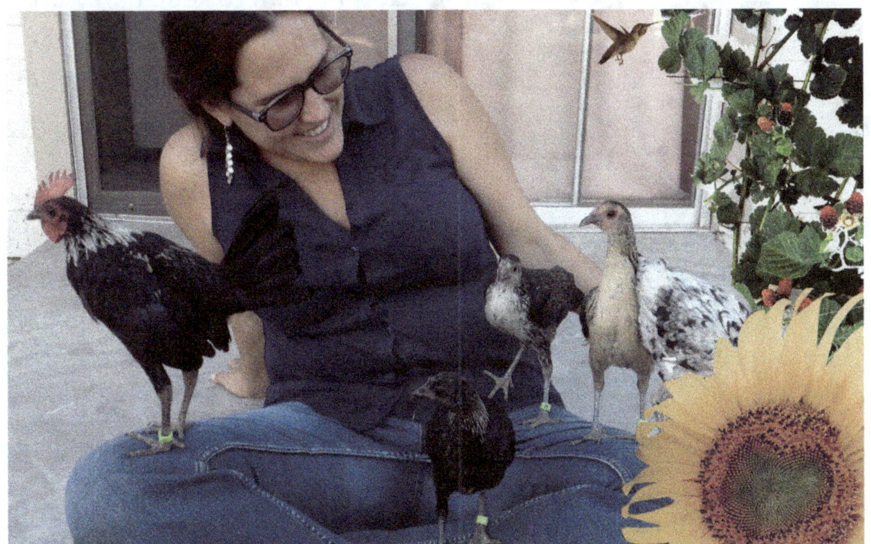

We would talk for hours about the two babies we wanted, a boy and a girl. We imagined our children's personalities, how sweet and beautiful they would be, and even chose names.

One day, our dream came true. I gave birth to our first child, a son, in 2017.

Usually, a pregnancy is from thirty-eight to forty-two weeks. With our son, I started contractions at twenty-seven weeks; he arrived at thirty-five weeks. His arrival was unusual.

We lived in a small town then. The hospital had a new labor and delivery wing but no neonatal intensive care unit (NICU). When they saw our baby would be premature, they smartly flew us by helicopter to a larger, well-equipped hospital. Thankfully, our healthy son did not need a NICU.

Following his birth, my husband's and my anxiety levels were high. Disinformation online about how chickens, gardens, and even dirt could harm my child only intensified my anxiety.

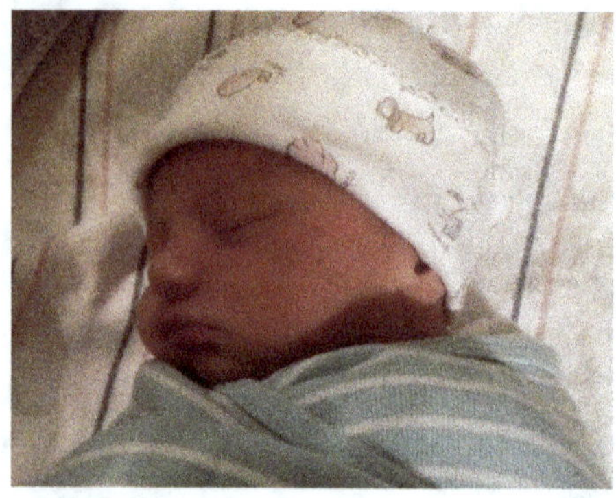

My son was tiny and skinny, so it was hard to keep his temperature at a healthy level. I remembered double clothing him to keep him warm. And because he was born premature, I stayed with him until he reached a healthy weight.

Dealing with the hormonal and emotional changes that come with pregnancy was challenging. I rarely slept or showered during the first two months following his birth. I would breastfed him, and then after feeding, I would burp him and change his diaper. Soon after, I would have to do it all again. He slept in my arms those first weeks; I held him, talked to him, and touched him; we bonded.

Our son was my world, and I feared something would happen to him. I would not let him out of sight, and because my son dominated my life, I forgot about caring for myself and my marriage. My husband and I started to disconnect.

My husband struggled too, with his inner conflicts. Our lives drastically changed shortly after our son's birth when we had to move. Giving away and selling the diminutive hen pets he had hatched and reared into adults broke his heart and sent him into a dark place. It did not help to leave behind the cherished garden we so lovingly tended. We looked for other ways to replace what we had lost.

One day, he asked if I would like to move to Wisconsin. We had visited friends who lived there months before in summertime and fell in love with the state. We decided we wanted a fresh start, a new adventure. Now was a perfect time. We were an energetic, healthy, and young family. We left the option open to return to California if we changed our minds. My husband, a talented service technician for air-conditioning and heating units, could easily find work. We moved from California to Wisconsin one year after our son's birth.

Our friends helped us until we found a beautiful studio apartment in a home across from a park next to a lake. I loved Wisconsin, the people, and the seasonal changes.

The season's changes were something I'd never before experienced. Seasonal changes in the Midwest were more distinct than in Southern California and Peru.

My favorite season was fall. I loved when the tree leaves turned red, orange, and yellow. I loved spring when the weather started warming; the trees and plants blossomed, and everything turned green. Summer was wet and beautiful. Chasing those amazing fireflies was a new experience. I never had enough of watching them flicker about on humid nights.

Even though wintertime was beautiful, I cannot say I liked winter. Nor did I have much experience with snow. I became anxious in winter when the days were shorter and overcast, and

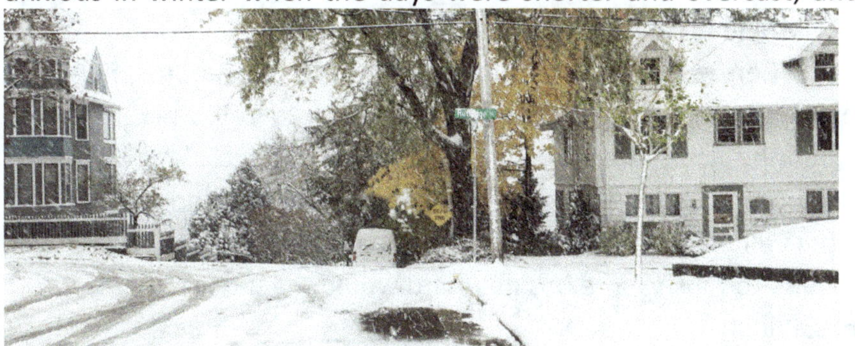

sunlight was scarce.

A cold December day in 2019, I finished a tiring work day at the daycare center my two-year-old son also attended. On this day, I did not have the patience I usually have while caring for these children. While I buckled my son into his car seat, I started crying. My emotions were chaotic. I listened to rhythm and blues to calm down and thought about how I felt: tired, emotional, and agitated. "Could I be pregnant?" I thought.

I stopped at the pharmacy on the way home to buy a pregnancy test. I checked once I arrived home and learned I was pregnant. This discovery was exciting yet scary and confusing. A follow-up appointment with my primary doctor confirmed my pregnancy.

My husband and I dreamed of having a second child, yet so much was happening. I had just started this fantastic job, but we struggled to keep our marriage together. Since the move, we had separated twice but kept working on our relationship.

The weather was cooling, and my husband said snow would soon follow. I remembered that I had postpartum depression with my son. Furthermore, here I was in a city with which I had not yet become familiar and with apprehension over a rapidly approaching winter.

Because my first pregnancy was not easy, I had many questions. Can I care for this baby and our two-year-old son? Will this baby be premature, like our firstborn? What if I develop postpartum depression as I did with our firstborn? I felt overwhelmed and started having panic attacks.

Before I found out I was pregnant the second time, my husband and I had discussed moving back to California. However, when the panic attacks began, I quit my job and told my husband I wanted to move before winter arrived. My father and brother flew from California and drove our son and me back. My husband stayed behind to finish some business and would meet us as soon as possible.

Part Two
The Pregnancy

I immediately contacted my OB/GYN to start prenatal care.

This pregnancy was unlike my first one. When I was ten weeks pregnant, I started cramping and saw spots of bright red blood in my underwear. I did not want to believe this was happening. To keep me from falling apart, my mind told me I imagined the cramps and blood drops. It was a weekend, so I went to the hospital emergency room.

The emergency room staff saw the hCG numbers had dropped and sent me home.

"Stay off your feet and rest," they said. "If you experience cramping and more bleeding, return to the emergency room."

I experienced more bleeding the next day and returned to the busy emergency room. Thinking about what could happen scared me. The emergency room staff performed an ultrasound. The baby looked okay, but the hCG numbers were still dropping. They told me there was nothing they could do.

"Go home," the doctor said. "Go home and rest because you may lose your baby. Call your primary doctor in the morning, but return to the emergency room if anything changes."

What the ER doctor said tore me up inside. I called my aunt, a doctor who explained what was happening to me in plain terms. "Your body will know, Nathalia; it could happen when you go to the bathroom."

Crying and in shock, I thought, "I cannot believe it! I do not want to consider it!"

I did not tell my husband because he was out of town. It would be a few days before he came home, and I did not want to give him the news while he was driving.

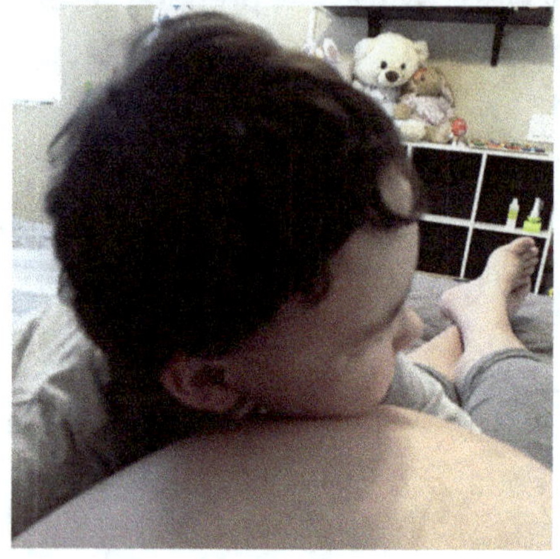

That night, I stayed in my room with my son. I remember curling up and feeling lost. Even though I was not feeling well, I would not break down in front of my son. My sister-in-law told me about a mother going through the same issues. This story kept me from falling apart because that baby was fine.

On the following Monday, my OB/GYN saw me. He performed an ultrasound and heard the baby's strong heartbeat. "Sometimes, those numbers drop when you are around 10-11 weeks pregnant. It is normal for that to happen," he said. His words eased my anxiety. Finally, I could breathe.

At my sixteen-week appointment, my doctor and I discussed the possibility of postpartum depression, depression that occurs after the birth of a baby. I had postpartum depression with our first child. In my doctor's experience, postpartum depression with a second child is usually worse than with the first.

COVID-19 was in its early stages, and my doctor's concern was premature delivery. He wanted to be sure about this pregnancy, so he sent me to a genetic specialist. "The specialist checks the baby for any complications using an ultrasound and gives an okay to start with progesterone," my doctor explained.

I remember doing the ultrasound with my son because I refused the blood test for Down syndrome. It did not matter if he had Down syndrome because I would accept him either way. The ultrasound took about an hour and a half because they measured every bone and organ.

"If the specialist agrees you need progesterone, you will see me for the progesterone injection, then return to the specialist. They will perform an ultrasound, measure the baby, measure the cervix for dilation, and then check how the baby responded to the progesterone."

"What is progesterone," I asked.

"Your body naturally makes this hormone but may not produce enough," he said.

"Progesterone is a steroid hormone that protects the fetus and prepares the body for birth."

A new nurse performed the ultrasound during one visit with the specialist and had difficulty getting a 3D image. She handed me the pictures and asked me to wait for the specialist. I thought the photos were not as clear compared with the ones before.

I thought, "Why couldn't she get a good image? Maybe the nurse did not know how to use the machine."

When the specialist arrived, he checked the nurse's notes, looked at the screen, and, just like that, said, "Your baby may have Down syndrome or achondroplasia." He never looked at me as he closely examined the nurses' notes.

I sat behind him, shocked and confused by his explanation. I asked, "Ako, what? What do you mean? The baby was perfect on our last visit." I had no idea what he was talking about.

He looked at the nurse's notes. "The humerus bone, the long bone of the upper arm, and the femoral bone of the upper leg are five weeks behind in growth and are not growing normally. That is one sign." He patiently explained why he measured the length and shape of long bones (*Altman, 2002*).

"Are you sure about these results? Are the measurements on those blurred pictures correct?" I asked anxiously. It frightened me to think something was not right with my baby.

He checked the ultrasound photos. "Yes, they are blurry." He then looked at the old ultrasound and pointed, "Look, you can see the forehead is prominent here, and the hand is a trident shape. The fingers are the same size," he calmly explained. "They deviate and give the hand a starfish shape."

Our beautiful baby looked like she was waving at me or doing

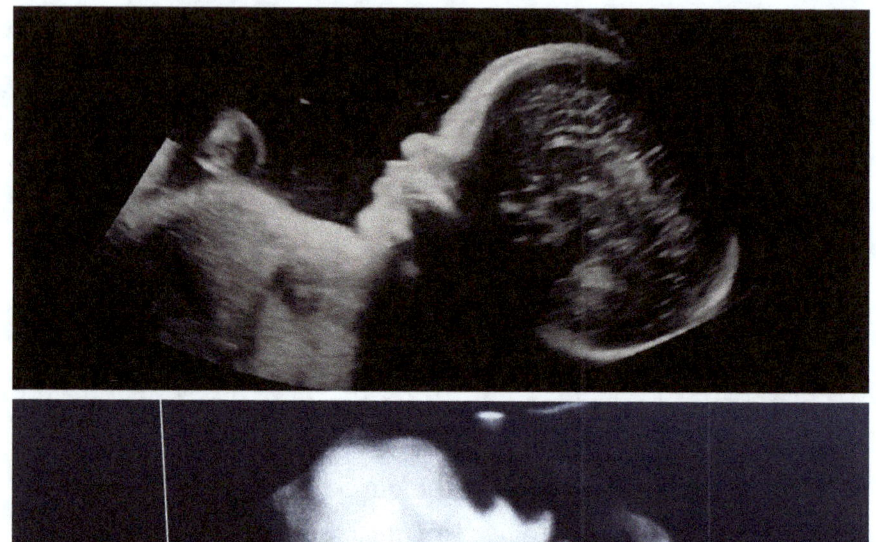

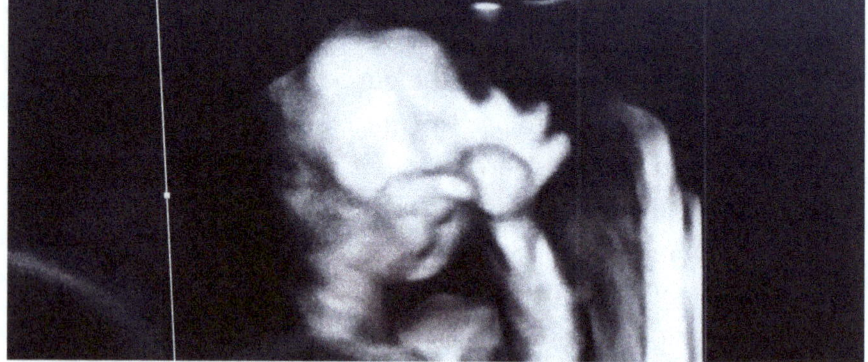

high-fives.

"Looks more like achondroplasia. Something is going on with your baby," he said.

"Ako, what?" I asked again.

He talked about a famous actor in a movie and said our baby was like that. I do not remember if he said The Lord of The Rings or Game of Thrones. I asked him to write the name of the diagnosis on a piece of paper because I had no idea which actor he was talking about. My world was spinning.

The doctor clarified, "A mutation came from you or your husband. Neither of you did anything wrong; it just happens, and we can do nothing to prevent it."

The next plan was to do a blood test for Down syndrome. The blood test was not 100% certain, but I did it because it was simple.

"There is a test to check for achondroplasia called amniocentesis," he explained. "We remove a sample of amniotic fluid from the uterus for testing. With this test comes a risk of infection and a chance for premature delivery."

I decided not to do that test and risk our baby's life because nothing could change the diagnosis. I did not know anyone who knew anything about achondroplasia. I did not know anyone who could explain it to me. I could not even pronounce the name. I worried I would lose her. The doctor agreed with me and scheduled an ultrasound in a month.

While waiting, I researched achondroplasia (*Children's Hospital of Philadelphia*) and found it is the most common type of disproportionate dwarfism, a genetic condition affecting bones and cartilage. According to the American Academy of Pediatrics, two to five percent of babies with achondroplasia die from central apnea due to compression of the brainstem and arteries without early intervention and assessment.

Researching more about achondroplasia only worsened my anxiety, so I stopped reading. I was in shock and prayed and asked God to protect our baby. I left the doctor's office more confused and scared than when I arrived.

"Our baby may be a little person," I told my husband. "But I do not feel the ultrasound is right."

My husband was supportive and encouraging. "If the baby does have dwarfism, she will be the most beautiful little person," he said. "Small and beautiful." I smiled and hugged him. We went home.

The following week, I went to my primary doctor appointment. We talked about what the specialist said, and I expressed my thoughts.

"Look," the doctor said. "You did nothing wrong and can do

nothing to change it. Until the baby arrives, we will not know anything 100%. So, relax and enjoy your pregnancy. Maybe the baby looks small because some Latin babies are small. It may be achondroplasia, but your baby will be okay, and you will love her, Nathalia."

His compassion and encouragement helped me feel better, so I returned home to wait for my next ultrasound. My family prayed that, the baby was okay.

While waiting for my next appointment, I prayed with my cousin, who was preparing to be a pastor. We prayed for my baby, for my depression not to resurface, and to guide the doctors. Praying helped me feel better because I knew God was protecting my baby.

*"Do not be anxious about anything, but in every
situation through prayer and petition, with thanksgiving,
present your requests to God, and the peace of God, which
transcends all understanding, will guard your hearts and
minds in Christ Jesus - Philippians 4:6-7*

At my next ultrasound appointment, the doctor again said that it looked more like our baby had achondroplasia. I did not worry because I knew God would care for her.

My mother cried when I told her. My dad said, "We will pray and leave it in God's hands." It scared my parents, not knowing. They worried about us, our daughter's life, and the possible medical complications.

Days later, I received a call from genetic specialists who wanted to discuss Down syndrome, achondroplasia, and any genetic problems. They confirmed she did not have Down's syndrome and asked if I wanted to keep my pregnancy.

"Are you asking me if I want to keep my baby?" I replied, shocked at her question. "What is wrong with people?" I am sure my tone of voice was angry. "Are you really asking me this? She is thirty-three weeks old. Do people have abortions for achondroplasia? Do people have abortions this late?"

She was silent. I imagined her question shamed her.

She replied, "Some people do, and some clinics are willing to do it." I said, "Not me! I love my baby. It does not matter if she has a genetic abnormality. I chose to keep my pregnancy. After the phone call, I felt angry and sad but knew I had two choices.

The first choice: I could talk and cry about the diagnosis, research achondroplasia, find out the worst-case scenarios, and make myself depressed. That would then affect my son, baby, and me and possibly affect postpartum depression. Who knows? What if she did have achondroplasia? What could I do to change the result? Nothing.

My second choice was to enjoy my pregnancy and recognize my son as an only child until our baby arrived.

I chose choice number two. I would enjoy my pregnancy.

COVID-19 frightened me. People stayed home, and my husband could not go with me to every doctor's visit because of the virus protocols. Nevertheless, I had appointments twice weekly, one for progesterone shots and the second with the specialist to check the baby and see if I was dilating.

I had started having contractions, and because of this, they had to check the baby's stress levels. The doctors noted those at each visit and added a third weekly appointment.

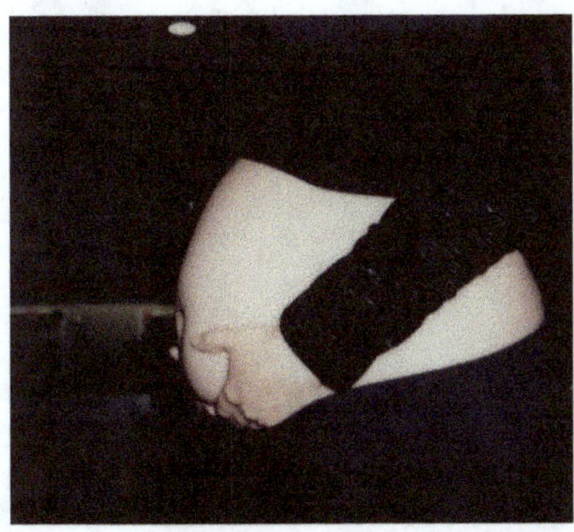

One day, after losing my balance and falling, I called my doctor. He checked the baby and me and said, "Your fall did not hurt either of you. Thanks to the extra fluid, the baby swam around in your belly. However, the baby is thirty-five weeks, and you measure forty weeks."

The genetic specialist recommended a cesarean or c-section.

Because of the baby's prominent head and the extra amniotic fluid, the fluid pressure would force her out and may leave her struggling for oxygen. "A c-section will be safer for you and your baby," he said.

Following the specialist's recommendation, my doctor and I made plans for a cesarean at thirty-seven weeks because of the extra amniotic fluid.

"We will keep her in as long as possible to prevent premature delivery. This extra fluid is risky for the baby," he said. "Take it easy, do not drive, and do not go anywhere alone. If your water breaks, call 9-1-1 and try to hold the baby in because the amniotic fluids might force the baby and umbilical cord out. This is dangerous for you and the baby."

During my last appointment, I asked my doctor, "Do you think the progesterone shots created the extra amniotic fluids? Could they be hurting the baby?" I knew nothing about how genetic abnormalities developed and naively thought that progesterone affected my daughter's growth.

"No," he said. "The progesterone is not producing the extra amniotic fluids, but having a baby with a genetic diagnosis normally causes extra fluids."

"I am still having many contractions," I said.

"The extra fluid," he said, "allows the baby to move around more, and the baby moving causes you to have more contractions."

My contractions became hard during the night. My husband drove me to the hospital, where the doctor admitted me. Our baby was on her way.

Part Three
The Birth

July 21, 2020. My husband and I drove to the hospital, where the doctor admitted me. We had not had time to reserve a room for the c-section, but they found me a room because of my circumstances. Our baby was on her way—finally, an open space.

I was in a private room in the maternity ward. The nurses checked the baby and me frequently with the fetal heart monitor.

Our son FaceTimed me often because it was our first time apart in his three years of life. What a frightening experience.

An epidural block is a procedure where doctors inject anesthesia into the epidural space of the spinal cord. The purpose is to provide a lack of feeling in certain body parts.

The anesthesiologist injected anesthesia into the lower part of my back so I would not feel anything during the c-section, but I would still be awake.

The following afternoon, the operating room staff prepared me for an epidural block (*Healthline, 2021*). The medication worked as it traveled and numbed my legs and feet. I wanted to scratch my legs but could not move, and because I could not move, I became anxious as excitement overwhelmed us.

Before our child's birth, we had not discussed the possibility of achondroplasia and spoke only that we would soon hold our precious baby girl in our arms. I could barely contain my excitement now that our dream of having a second child was coming true. How happy our son would be to meet his younger sister.

They placed a screen in front of my face and across my chest so we could not see the doctors performing the surgery.

I remember feeling like they were doing something invasive and then sudden relief---I heard our baby's cries. My heart swelled, and I tightly squeezed my husband's hand.

The nurse called my husband to see his newborn daughter. They brought our daughter from around the screen to me. Seeing her for the first time was a wonderfully surreal feeling, knowing that I held her in my belly for months and felt her kick and move around as she grew.

Now, I could not hold her or touch her. They did not place

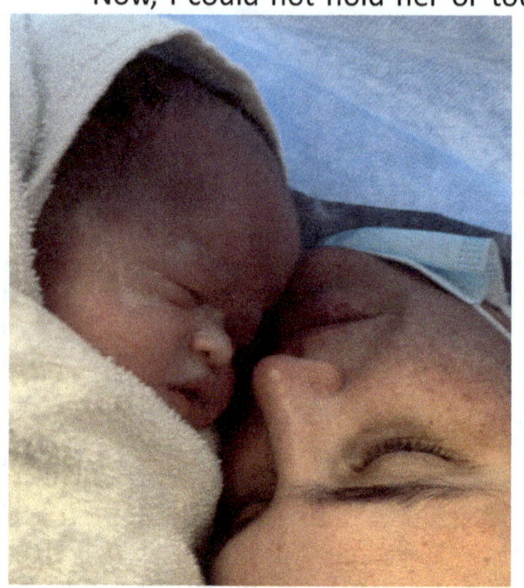

her on my chest like my firstborn but allowed me to kiss her soft, warm face. Still feeling the effects of anesthesia, I thought they would bring her back to me after closing the incision, but they did not. Everything happened quickly; my husband accompanied her to the NICU. Soon, I was in my room resting, but I still could not see our baby. "Where is my baby?" I asked. "She is in the NICU," the nurse replied. "You will see her soon."

Much later, my husband came into the room. He looked exhausted. He looked like he was ready to explode. "I need a break," he said breathlessly. "I saw your parts next to you on the table," he exclaimed, pacing.

"What do you mean?" I asked.

"Your internal organs were sitting outside you. No one warned me not to look. They just called me over. And then, this doctor took me to a small room and told me our daughter had achondroplasia. He told me about all the frightening health problems that went with it and said so many scary things could happen to her that I could not understand." They just threw everything at me, Nathalia."

I felt terrible for my husband. We had never had a serious conversation about the possibility of our baby having achondroplasia. We had not discussed it before because we wanted to enjoy the pregnancy. Moreover, he could not go with me to my appointments because of COVID-19.

Before her birth, I could not tell him about our baby's possible condition because I was unsure; I did not want to frighten him. It shocked and scared me, too. I thought not talking or thinking about it would protect me from postpartum depression and allow me to enjoy my pregnancy.

Because my husband struggled with chronic depression, I shielded him from the unpleasant potential health problems. Thinking that something could happen to our children scared him. However, before he could even enjoy the experience of our new daughter, the doctors showered him with information about her condition. He then learned about her diagnosis and the unpleasantness of potential health problems. He endured all this alone. I could not be by his side to tell him everything would be okay.

"Where is the baby?" I asked him.

"I walked with her to the NICU," he said. "I carried her, and then they took her from me. She is beautiful, Nathalia. But they are working on her, putting all these tubes and wires in her," he said again while pacing. "I need some air." He walked outside. He was not doing well at all, and hospitals scared him.

As soon as he left, the genetics doctor came in and introduced himself. He appeared upset that my husband had gone on break. I do not know if he sensed our anxiety or what we were going through.

"He went outside to take a break," I said. The doctor's abrupt manner bothered me, but his voice had a sense of urgency and conciseness when he spoke about our daughter.

The doctor said, "I will tell you about the achondroplasia trial studies. It is an important study about achondroplasia appropriate for your daughter's age. Someone from the dysplasia clinic will contact you on a video call." I knew the information he gave me was essential to our daughter's health. I told him I still had not seen my daughter but wanted to learn everything related to her and her diagnosis. Then, a nurse entered the room carrying a laptop. "You have a Zoom call," she said. A female doctor appeared on the screen and introduced herself. We talked about the achondroplasia trial. She explained, "I am not part of this study but am interested because I work with many children in the dysplasia clinic. Dysplasia is an abnormal growth of tissue or cells."

She said, "Your daughter has achondroplasia. Her bones are smaller than an average infant's bones. Complications may develop. Her condition needs testing and, possibly, surgeries. These children are fragile, so you must care for your baby's head and neck. These children have bigger heads. An abnormality of the spine called kyphosis causes a curvature of the upper back, which causes pain and stiffness."

She threw information at me fast and spoke in choppy sentences, but I sensed the urgency. Scared, I explained that I had an energetic toddler. "Will she be fragile around him?"

She replied, "For example, a mother was in bed with her baby, and the little brother came in and jumped on the bed. The results were tragic."

She must have read the fear on my face because she quickly added, "Girls do better than boys."

She said if my daughter does not get into the study, the insurance may refuse to pay for the needed medication. This medication helps children with achondroplasia and may prevent some medical complications associated with abnormal skeletal growth.

She ended the conversation with one last piece of advice, "Once the hospital discharges your daughter, make a follow-up appointment with a geneticist at the dysplasia clinic. Genetic doctors' appointments book quickly. Contact the people for the study if you are interested because there are not many open spaces for your daughter's age, so do this soon. I know you will have many questions, as most parents do." And just like that, the video call ended.

The hospital genetic doctor asked for a blood test to confirm our baby's achondroplasia diagnosis.

My mind was blank yet overflowing with information and questions. I asked to see my child because I had not seen her in many hours. The nurse wheeled me in a wheelchair to the NICU. Before entering the NICU, the nurses gave me a code to get into the room and a special robe and showed me how to wash my hands antiseptically.

I saw my baby in bed with intravenous medications, oxygen, and a tube taped to her face. The sight was emotionally overwhelming; she looked so fragile that she could break any moment. I told her I loved her, held her hand, and kissed her.

I barely breath. She looked frail and helpless, swaddled in a

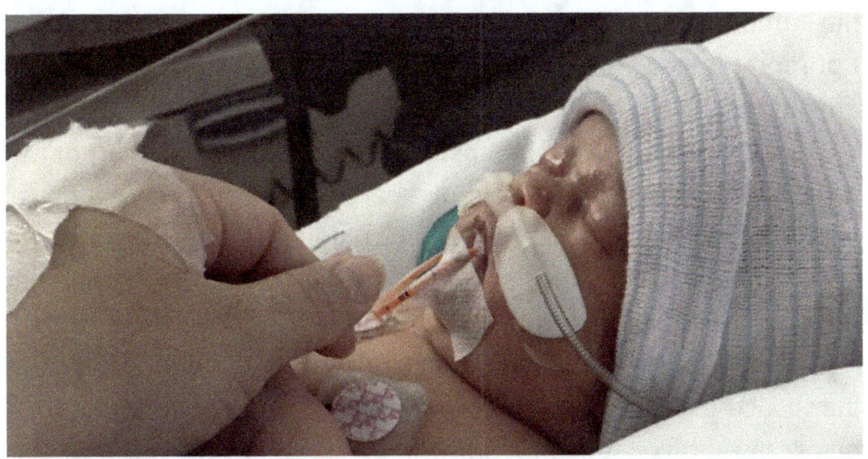

bassinet away from other babies. She had been next to my heart for thirty-six and a half weeks. Now, I wondered if everything would be okay.

A cacophony of sounds from beeping machines and activated alarms echoed off the walls of the cold room. Notes taped to the wall above her said how fragile she was. I did not want to break down beside her, so the nurse wheeled me back to my room. I sat in silence alone while my mind raced. I had many questions but could not allow postpartum depression to happen!

I thought about my son being far away from me. My parents cared for him while my husband and I stayed with our daughter. It was hard to explain to him what was happening with his sister.

How long can she live like this? I would want to die with her. Fear and worry overwhelmed me, thinking she would die without giving us a chance to bond with her as I did with our son. I could not hold or breastfed her, and COVID-19 restrictions further limited my time with our children. This horrible separation left me with an empty and sad feeling.

I took a slow, deep breath. "I have to keep going," I told myself, so I called my parents and son. Because of coronavirus restrictions, they could not be with me. I sent a group text to my siblings. We cried together. I felt lost and alone.

The nurses were kind and patient and bottle-fed her and gave her antibiotics through an umbilical catheter in her belly button. I pumped breast milk to feed her. "Every three hours," the nurse encouraged.

While a patient in the hospital, I had access in and out of the NICU. The hospital's rules were one parent at a time and no siblings allowed. My husband visited the NICU alone. He felt helpless, not knowing how to help her—seeing her with all the tubes attached to her and not knowing what might happen frightened him.

I told myself, "You cannot do much for her right now except pump all the milk you can." I knew how vital mother's milk was for a baby's immune system and mother/child bonding. My purpose was to pump, pump, pump.

I pumped milk and took it to her, touched her, and sat beside her. Her pain was mine. I wanted to breastfed and bond with her, but I could not because of the many lines attached to her frail body.

The nurses said that her oxygen levels might drop if I breast-fed. I feared the unknown.

However, no matter how much I pumped, I was not generating enough milk—not having her next to me while pumping felt odd.

I went to the NICU and took a video of my daughter. I returned to my room and resumed pumping while watching the video. A miracle occurred. It confirmed how connected she was to me.

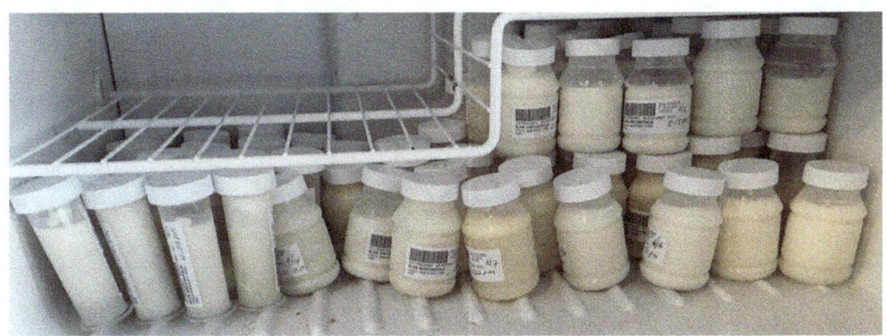

The milk poured from my breast. I pumped more than she needed and started her milk bank. I pumped milk daily, visited her in the NICU, and talked to her. The amount of milk I produced impressed the nurses.

I entered the hospital many days ago, pregnant with a baby.

What an empty and sad feeling when I left the hospital without my baby. My heart ached for her. I was thankful she was alive but felt like I had abandoned her. But my son, who filled my heart with hugs and kisses, kept me going.

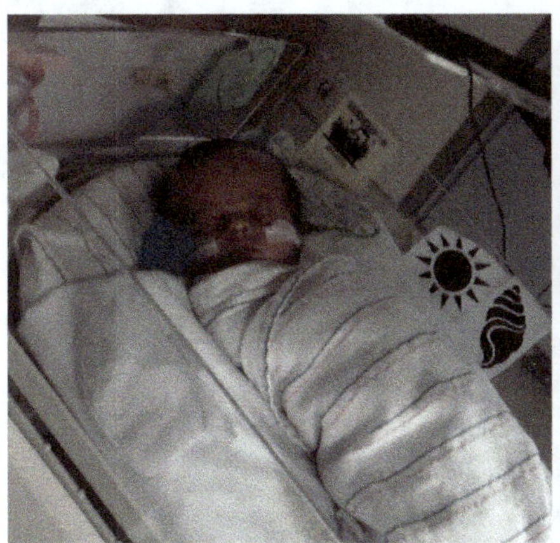
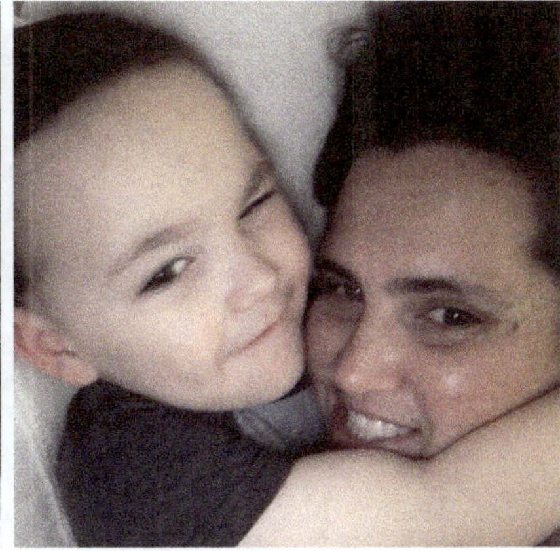

Part Four
Introducing Our Daughter

Because of our large families, COVID-19, and the distance we lived from each other, we could not easily visit one another, so we talked on the phone and by family group text.

Hello Family. We hope everyone is doing well. Our girl is stable and doing well; we hope she can return home soon.

She has achondroplasia, a type of dwarfism. This diagnosis has many health complications, is not going to be an easy journey but with love and acknowledgment everything will be okay.

Maybe you do not know what to say or how to feel. These feelings are normal. I have dealt with this possibility since I was twenty-nine weeks pregnant and could not believe it. Doctors told me again at thirty-three weeks; still, I did not embrace it. You never know until the baby's birth.

After her birth, I did not realize it until hours later when the doctors started talking to me about achondroplasia. She is in the NICU with some health complications associated with achondroplasia.

Achondroplasia is a mutation that can happen to anyone. It is most common in average-height parents and occurs once every 28,000 births. Amazing, ah? Achondroplasia is not just short stature. Achondroplasia babies may have complications affecting the spine and may face many surgeries.

Please feel free to ask questions or express any concerns you or my nieces and nephews may have. We must learn about her diagnosis; we cannot place our girl

*in a bubble. We will find a balance between caring for her
and letting her live her life. She may have difficulty
adjusting to the average-height world, but we will deal
with it together on her own time and in her own way.*

*I hope her diagnosis is just that she is a little person
with no health complications.*

Their responses were filled with love. I could see that my daughter has earned a special place in everyone's heart.

After learning about her diagnosis, I joined achondroplasia and dwarfism groups on Facebook. I wanted to collect as much information as possible. I emailed a mother with an achondroplasia child and another to two young women with achondroplasia. I pushed myself to learn everything I could to protect and fight for her because everything was different and new. With everyone's support, I believed everything would be okay.

I placed this next post on Facebook following the birth of our daughter. I wanted to open as many doors as possible for our baby girl, thank everyone for their prayers, and officially present her.

*We proudly present our beautiful daughter to you!
On Wednesday, July 22, 2020, at 4:30 p.m., our daughter
made her unscheduled appearance. She arrived at
thirty-six and a half weeks after a complicated pregnancy
followed by a cesarean.*

*I was lucky to kiss her before the nurses rushed her
to the NICU. She needed a little help.*

*Leaving the hospital without her was
heartbreaking, but I am grateful she is alive and receiving
good care.*

*Imagine there is one child out of 28,000 children
born with achondroplasia, and God chose us to be the
parents of this beautiful angel.*

*Our daughter is a fighter. Days after her birth, she
recognized me. Nurses swaddled her in a baby blanket so*

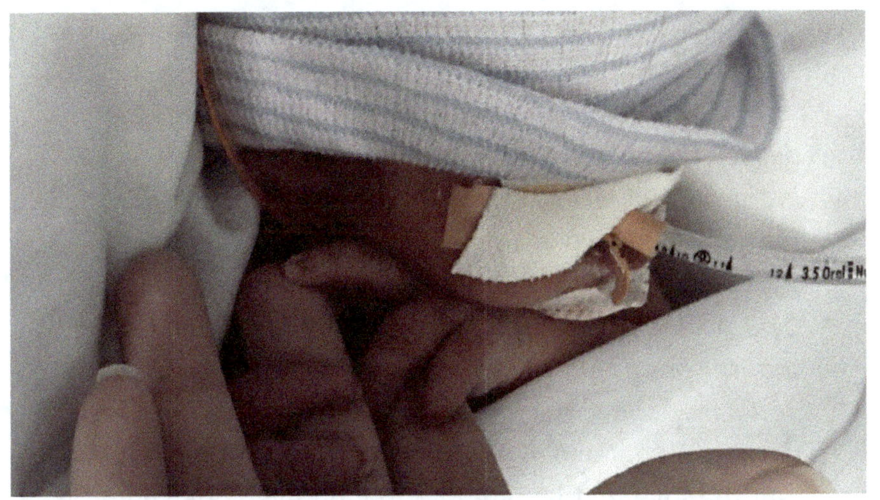

she could not move her hands and pull at the IV lines and other attachments. She struggled to escape confinement when she felt my presence nearby and grabbed my finger. I am overwhelmed with fear and excitement.

My daughter, I cannot wait for you to meet your older brother. One day, we will see you together, an average-height brother and little sister fighting together for a better world.

I garnered attention from this post. I have never had this many comments and likes during my Facebook time.

Commentaries from Peru, the United States, and Canada prayed for us and asked how she was doing. I knew that we had a mission in this world. So began my journal.

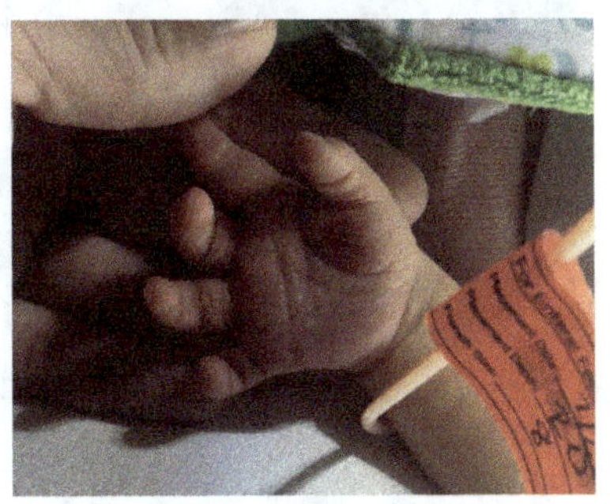

The blood results returned, and I learned about the discovered gene alteration. The FGFR3 gene is the only gene associated with achondroplasia, and since our daughter had this gene, we now knew for sure she had achondroplasia.

I learned to speak for her while she was in NICU. With so

many questions and concerns about her health and safety, I went on the online group chats and introduced myself.

I began. "I am new to this group. One week ago, I delivered a baby girl born with achondroplasia. She is still in the NICU. I feel lost because achondroplasia is new to me. I have many questions.

What do I need for her? Any recommendations on a particular crib, car seat, or stroller? The doctors tell me that she has fragile bones. I am afraid I may hurt her. How do I know I have a good doctor? It scares me that most doctors are unfamiliar with achondroplasia. Please help!"

All the love and helpful information everyone shared were tremendous blessings. I learned that babies with achondroplasia are stronger than most people think and that I was not alone on this journey.

With each visit, I saw our daughter's strength and confidence grow. She would recognize my voice and struggle out of her wrap to grab and cling to my finger. She would smile at me, and I knew she

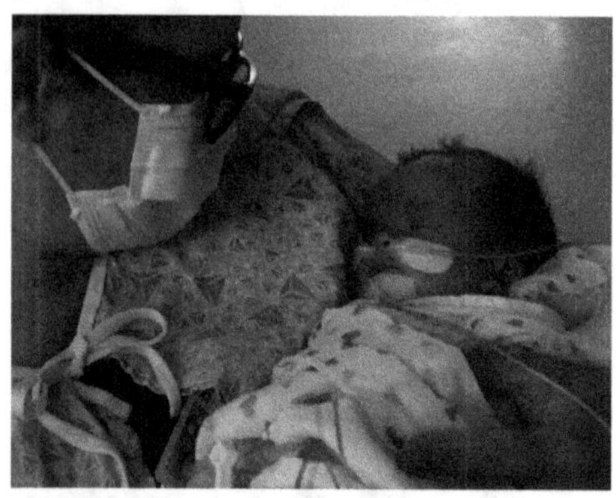

felt safe when I was nearby. She gave me the strength to keep going.

The first time I carried her, I had so much back pain that my body shook, and I was frightened that I might hurt her. She looked up at me with a big smile as if to say, "Hey, I am okay." I was so in love with her.

I was taking a more active role in her care and had a problem.

I asked the group, "How do I change diapers? The NICU therapists told me not to put her legs up when changing her diaper because she is fragile. It is not good for her back," they said.

"It frightened me today when a nurse pulled her

legs up to change her diaper. When they said it harmed the baby, I asked why she did it that way. She replied, 'The therapist said it was okay to change her this way.'"
Caring for our daughter was a learning experience for everyone.

Each day passed slowly, and she was still receiving oxygen, struggling with jaundice, and receiving antibiotics for an infection. They were working on lowering her oxygen intake, but her oxygen saturation levels were unstable and even dropped with bottle feeding.

She stayed in a NICU incubator with unique lights to treat neonatal jaundice (*Very well family*).

Finally, her jaundice and infection cleared, and her oxygen intake and saturation levels were at a manageable level. A doctor approached me and said, "Your baby is ready to go home."

"No," I said. "I cannot go home; she is wearing oxygen!" I wanted to go home, but I wanted to be sure that this was safe for her. I felt they did not understand my concerns and thought I was a mother with a hormonal imbalance who did not accept her baby's diagnosis. I learned from the online groups that babies with achondroplasia need baseline testing in the first months of life, an MRI to check for cervical spine compression, and a sleep study to check for apnea.

The doctor replied, "The clinician from the dysplasia clinic said we would not do the testing here. Once we discharge her, they will test at the dysplasia clinic in her follow-up appointment."

"Yes," I said. "But that would only happen if there were no complications and she left the hospital within five days following delivery." I had read that five to eight percent of achondroplasia babies can die from compression apnea. That was my trigger for pushing for the testing.

Stress overwhelmed me with my concerns about our daughter's condition, and pumping my breasts every three hours with very little sleep was too much. I stopped pumping my breast because I had developed mastitis, an infection of the breast tissue that causes pain, swelling, warmth, and redness. I believe there were many contributing factors to mastitis. One big reason was postpartum stress. Going to the NICU to see our daughter and then returning home to care for our energetic son was difficult. My active son had many questions about his sister and worried I was not with him as much. "Mommy, where are you?" He would ask when I was away. "Where is my sister? Where are you going? When are you coming home?"

Another factor was concern over her care. Because every day, we had new nurses who knew nothing about achondroplasia but were willing to learn. My daughter's oxygen saturation continued to drop with her feeding. Maternal instinct told me something was wrong. I did not want to transfer her to the nearby children's hospital because I felt uncomfortable with that clinic and did not want to drive her while she was on oxygen.

"She is ready to go home, and she is going with oxygen," the doctors insisted. "We have a plan for you and your daughter to spend a day in one of our rooms. This will allow you to get comfortable feeding her and using the oxygen machine."

I thought about this plan and reluctantly agreed, "Okay." I felt trapped and knew I had to make a decision. I still felt uncomfortable driving her in my car to the clinic without knowing

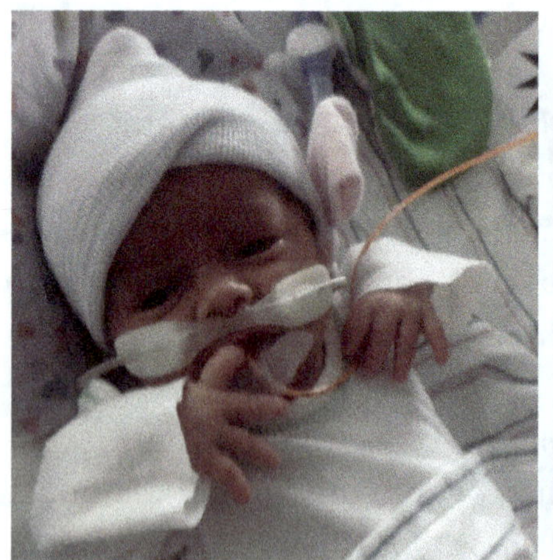
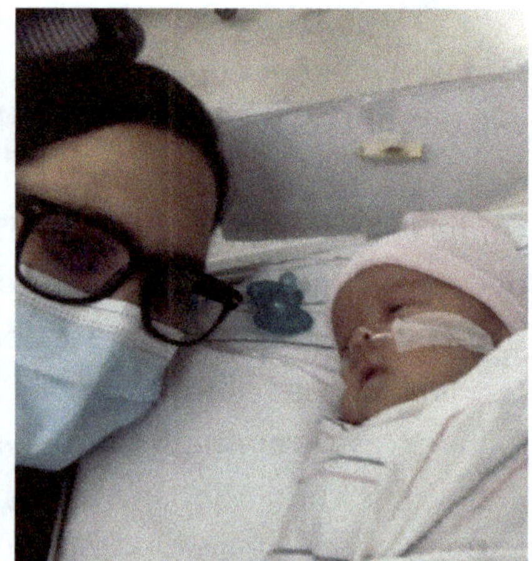

the root cause of why she was on oxygen.

Everything was okay while we were alone. She fed well, and I started to feel more comfortable.

At the day's end, her oxygen level began to drop when she received her last bottle. She looked at the top of my head and held her breath until her lips turned purple. She felt lighter. The machines started beeping louder and louder.

I gently stimulated her many times to get her back. Then, her oxygen level slowly began returning to normal. A nurse entered the room, and I explained what happened."

"That is not the first time this happened," the nurse said.

Because of this episode, my daughter remained in the NICU for five days. She could leave the NICU if she did not have an attack during that time.

Two days later, she had another apnea episode while sleeping. The machines started beeping and screaming while the nurses rushed in to help. I was not there when this happened, but the nurse explained what occurred when I called to check on my daughter.

When she had no more apnea episodes, a doctor approached me one day and said, "Your baby is ready to go home. "It is normal for kids to go home on oxygen; babies should be home with their mothers."

"I cannot take her home without an MRI and sleep study," I said. "You cannot tell me it is normal for her to go home with oxygen without knowing why she needs it. She cannot go home without answers!" I pleaded.

For forty-four days, our daughter stayed in the NICU. No tests were performed, no MRI and no sleep study, the doctors felt the problem was me not accepting our daughter's diagnosis.

I started researching her chart because they were not telling me everything but they told me that everything going on with her was in her file.

"I want to meet with the medical staff caring for my

daughter," I said, speaking with the NICU head doctor after reading my child's chart. I felt that no one was listening to me. "I will not take her home until we know what is happening with her. I want her transferred to a different hospital."

"Okay," he agreed. "I will plan a meeting with the NICU personnel."

I walked into a conference room full of medical personnel the following day. They sat in a circle and left one empty chair for me. I felt intimidated when I looked around the room and recognized the medical personnel caring for my child.

I recognized the doctors who had attended to our daughter, the nursing supervisor, the head of the NICU, accounting, an occupational therapist, and a couple more. They waited for me to sit down and talk about her. I felt as though I was on trial.

"Thank you for what you are doing," I said, starting the conversation. "I want my daughter transferred to another hospital specializing in achondroplasia."

Before the meeting, I had emailed a geneticist and a neurosurgeon from the LPA medical board with her health history.

They worried about spinal/brainstem compression. They asked me to check her neck.

"My daughter needs more testing. I had read that two to five percent of babies with achondroplasia die from apnea due to compression of the upper end of the spinal cord. I have been unable to sleep since her first episode because I worry that she may die anytime."

I talked about how sleep apnea and spinal cord compression complicate the lives of children with achondroplasia and how they can lead to long-term damage. I spoke of the mothers I have talked to with achondroplasia babies. Spinal compression was the cause of similar complications as my daughter's, and surgery corrected the compression in these children.

I continued. "I gave birth to my daughter at this

hospital on July 22, 2020. She was born with achondroplasia. Achondroplasia affects one in 27,000 births. Most infants with achondroplasia do not need extra care at birth, but my daughter does. She has been in the NICU for over a month. For a short time, she needed a ventilator to help her breathe. Now, she uses oxygen to breathe. She has problems during feeding."

"After one month and a week in the NICU, she began to have the following episodes," I said, ticking off a list of symptoms.

"She held her breath until she felt lighter. Her oxygen saturation dropped to 60. Her oxygen dropped during feeding, and her lips turned purple. She stopped breathing while sleeping. A normal infant's heart rate is 120 bpm to 160 bpm. Her heart rate dropped to 100 one day and 47 the next day."

"Her episodes are getting worse, not better. This hospital does not have any specialists in achondroplasia. We must transfer her to a hospital specializing in achondroplasia so she can have proper testing and see a specialist knowledgeable about achondroplasia. Families come worldwide to see the specialists at these hospitals."

"Hydrocephalus, sleep apnea, and spinal compression complicate the lives of children with achondroplasia. We have to check for these problems immediately to prevent long-term damage."

"The American Academy of Pediatrics stated that unexpected infant deaths occur without aggressive evaluation. These deaths affect about 2% to 5% of all infants with achondroplasia".

"My daughter is getting worse. You can see that from her recent episodes. Every day that passes is critical for her life and for preventing future

complications." I explained.

The doctors agreed to help.

"We will call her insurance plan and transfer her," one doctor said to the NICU team and the insurance lady. This doctor called the hospital to arrange the transfer.

Both hospitals agreed to the transfer, but the insurance denied the coverage for ambulance transport. On the transfer notes, it did not show any emergency but said, "Baby with achondroplasia wants to transfer."

Everyone was understandably upset. The doctor approached me and said, "OK, she is ready to go home. It is up to you."

"No," I said, "she needs more testing. I did not go through all this to let her die at home in my bed."

"If I do the testing, will you go home?" He asked.

"No," I replied, "because you will need a specialist to read the tests."

They went ahead and performed an X-ray.

I talked with the manager of the NICU and explained my daughter's circumstances. I told her the ambulance transfer sheet showed this was not an emergency. I asked her for help to transfer her and let them know this was an emergency. She told me she would talk with the doctors.

While sitting there holding my daughter, my phone rang. The geneticist, who was in the hospital, wanted to meet.

Unknown to me, the geneticist, the NICU doctor, and the insurance representative had a meeting before calling me. They had hoped the geneticist could allay my fears about taking my daughter home.

"I thought you would be home by now," he said when I met him in the hospital.

"No," I said. "We are still here and have been here for five weeks. I am waiting to know why she is still here. She continues to have these apnea episodes, and they have done no tests."

He sounded surprised. "I was the one who told you about

your daughter when you first gave birth. I remember you."

"I remember you, too. You talked about her diagnosis so excitedly," I replied. "But you did not tell me why she was in the NICU."

This time, his concern was for her and me, not just her diagnosis. I understood his excitement because achondroplasia births are uncommon, and the focus of this study after her birth was important information he wanted to share.

"Please, help me transfer her to a hospital specializing in achondroplasia," I pleaded. "I am afraid she may have achondroplasia-related complications and needs a specialist."

"I see you have many questions that need answering. Let us transfer her," he said. He was genuinely sorry this had happened.

"The doctors wanted to send her to a nearby children's hospital, but I heard they had no beds," I said. "And I am not comfortable with that hospital."

I spoke with one mother who had guided me since my first post. She told me about a children's hospital two hours away. I called the insurance to confirm that they worked with this hospital and then spoke with the doctors to transfer us to this hospital.

Finally, the call I had been waiting for came in.

"Your insurance approved your daughter's transfer to the children's hospital," the caller said. "They also approved transport and will be here by helicopter or ambulance tonight."

I hugged my daughter and cried. "Thank you, God."

While I waited in the hospital, I held my crying daughter. She felt stiff; her neck felt stiff, and nothing I did could comfort her. A nurse beside me offered her help so I could go home and prepare for the trip.

When my son, mother and I returned to the hospital, I saw the ambulance and recognized the children's hospital logo. My heart swelled because a group entered the hospital; a medical team had arrived for my daughter.

I approached them and identified myself. "Are you here for

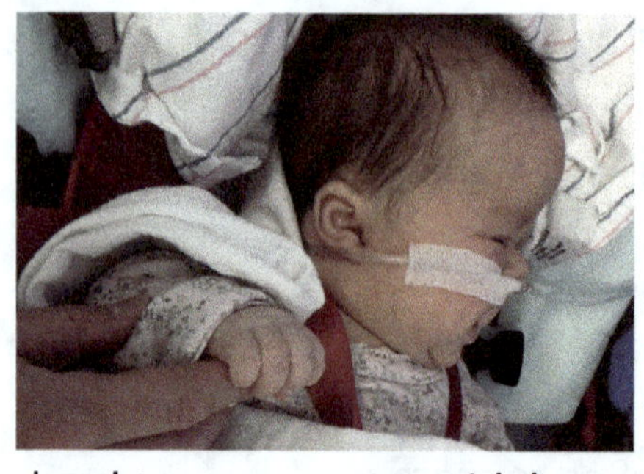

my daughter?"

"Yes," they said.

I replied, "We have been waiting for you."

They entered the NICU and collected all the information from the staff. They placed our daughter on a gurney with her oxygen and other machines to monitor her and loaded her into the ambulance.

My mother approached me when the children's hospital staff exited with my daughter. She was nervous and excited and asked if she could see the baby. The nurse said yes. Since her birth forty-four days ago, none of the family had seen her.

My mother burst into tears when she saw how fragile she looked on the gurney with her oxygen tube. "Nathalia, she is beautiful," she repeatedly said through tears. She was still crying while calling my dad to let him know.

After two hours, we arrived at the hospital. I placed our daughter in the hands of the specialists at the children's hospital. When the doctor first saw her, he asked, "Why is she wearing oxygen?"

After hearing the doctor ask this question, I knew she was in the right place.

That night, I slept soundly for the first time in months.

Part Five
Children's Hospital

After a good night's sleep, I returned to the hospital the following day. Our daughter had a private room with a security camera, so we could visit and stay overnight whenever possible. I checked her with the security monitor app when I left. This enabled me to spend time with my three-year-old son, who stayed with my mother and friends only minutes from the hospital.

Our daughter's team of doctors met every morning before rounds and talked about her case. They invited me to each meeting, and we spoke of her performance and activities of the previous day. They discussed their plans for her care and asked for my opinion. Each night, the team performed rounds to make sure she was okay for the night. The group believed I knew her better than anyone. I felt like I was part of her care team. I loved my daughter; her health and well-being were paramount.

The morning after her arrival, doctors wanted to discover why she needed oxygen. Technicians performed chest and spine X-rays, and a phlebotomist performed an arterial blood gas test (ABG).

Since she had apneic episodes, the ABG test assists in discovering her oxygen needs requirements.

> The ABG test measures blood oxygen and carbon dioxide levels. When you inhale and exhale, the lungs move oxygen into the blood and release carbon dioxide.

Following her x-rays and blood test, doctors scheduled an MRI, magnetic resonance imaging scan (*MRI-Mayo Clinic*), and a polysomnography or sleep study (*Morgan, 2021*) for the next day.

> The sleep study would show how long my daughter slept, total or partial breathing cessation, how many times she woke

The MRI of the head and neck would evaluate the foramen magnum. The foramen magnum is a large, oval-shaped opening in the skull's occipital bone (back of the head).

As they exit the skull, the brainstem and spinal cord pass through the foramen magnum.

The foramen magnum (*Vaughn, 2023*) is round in an average-height person. In someone with achondroplasia, the foramen magnum is smaller and shaped like an old fashioned keyhole where one end is wider than the other. This can lead to central apnea if the smaller end of the keyhole compresses the brainstem and spinal cord.

There are two types of apnea: obstructive apnea and central apnea.

Obstructive apnea (Mayo Clinic) is a disorder in which breathing stops because the throat muscles relax and block the airway. Obstructive apnea (*Sisk et al., 1999*) is the most common in children with achondroplasia because of their abnormally small airways within the nasal cavity and throat. Tonsils and adenoids blocking part of the airway can cause obstructive apnea. Surgical removal of tonsils and adenoids can improve breathing but is unnecessary in Central apnea.

Central apnea (Mayo Clinic) is a disorder in which breathing repeatedly stops and stars during sleep. Central sleep apnea occurs because the brain doesn't send proper signals to the muscles that control breathing. Central apnea (*Ratini, 2022*) is where compression or kinks at the foramen magnum in a child's

Parents and doctors of children with achondroplasia should watch out for the following symptoms: brisk reflexes, numbness, weakness, difficulty walking, loss of control of bowel and bladder, sleep apnea, or periods during sleep when breathing stops.

Gastroesophageal reflux (Mayo Clinic) can also cause obstructive apnea. However, with medication, a pulmonologist, gastroenterologist, or ENT (ear, nose, and throat) doctor may help eliminate this problem. My daughter had been on acid reflux medication since birth.

Our daughter had gastroesophageal reflux disease (GERD), common in babies with an achondroplasia diagnosis.

On September 10, our daughter underwent a sedated head,

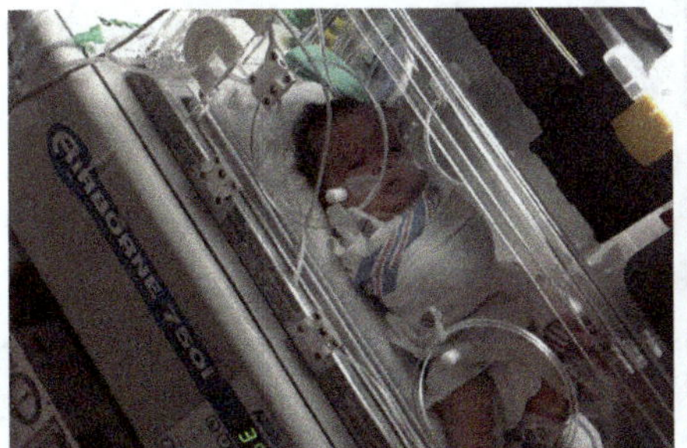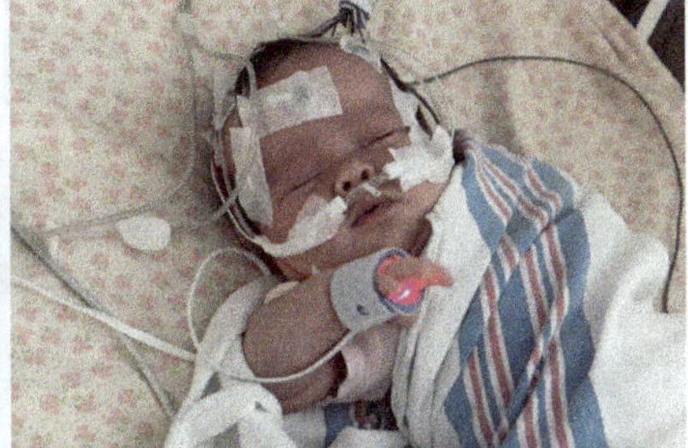

and spine MRI. When she returned, a sleep technologist performed a sleep study in the room while she napped.

The next day, the medical team arrived and showed me the test results. The MRI showed that she had severe compression of the brainstem at the foramen magnum (the narrow end of the keyhole) and needed decompressing surgery. The sleep study found central obstructive apnea secondary to the compression.

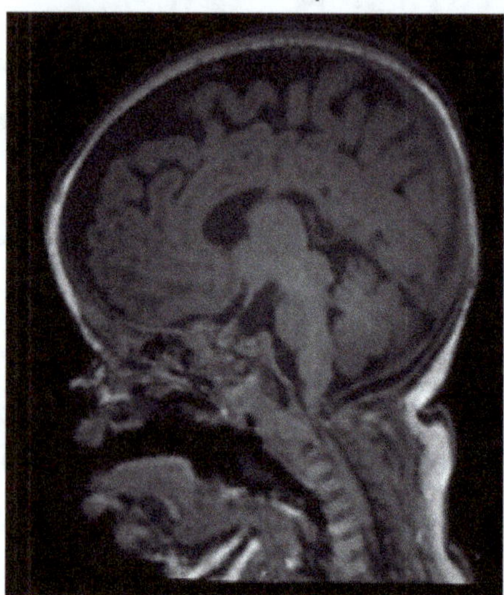
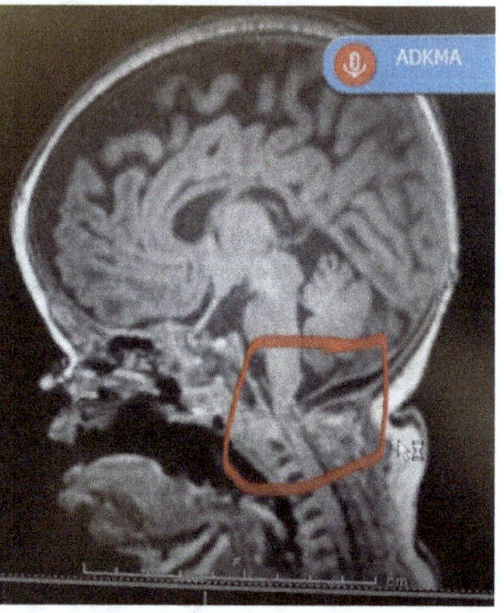

Our daughter suffered from complications typical of achondroplasia in babies, which could prove fatal if we overlooked and did not correct these issues.

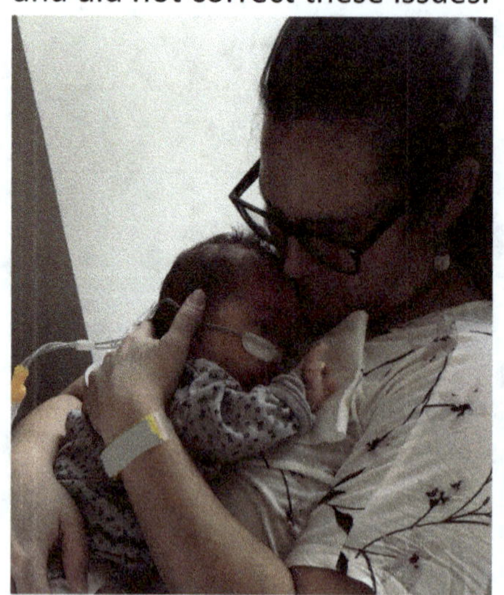

I spent our first night in the hospital and the night before her surgery with her. This was the first time she saw my face without the mask.

I held her, kissed her, sang to her, and repeatedly told her, "I love you." I could not cuddle with her often; somehow, I knew she felt safe and loved. She was so strong.

It frightened me that our

baby girl would undergo a delicate neck and head surgery. I imagined the possible complications of that surgery, and it broke my heart. She was not even two months old and had already gone through so much. Then, a neurosurgeon came into the room and allayed my fears. "Do not worry, We will be married on this" he said.

On September 14, a nurse arrived early to transfer her to the operation room and prepare her for decompression surgery. The surgeons would remove bone at the foramen magnum to relieve pressure on the spinal cord and brainstem. It was scary thinking about her going under anesthesia.

It is scary for any parent when their infant must undergo surgery and receive anesthesia.

> The risks for anesthesia in an infant with achondroplasia (*Spiegel, 2015*) are higher because their spinal cord is small, and they do not have a full range of motion in the joints. They have smaller tracheas that need great care when intubating. Unique positioning and head and neck support throughout surgery is vital because the bone structure here is not standard.

The anesthesiologist generally talks with the family before the surgery. This will give you time to ask questions and allay any fears about the surgery. I would therefore ask what experience they have working with achondroplasia in infants and would have information about the bones and joints of the neck of achondroplasia babies available for him.

Following my son's birth, I created an email account to send him letters of events and life experiences. Our son can read these letters as he grows older and reflect on his life. I also created an email account for our daughter following her birth. While in the waiting room, I wrote to her.

"My beautiful daughter," I wrote. "I am sitting in the waiting room while you are in surgery to decompress an area of your neck and spine. My nerves are killing me,

but I know you are in good hands, and God is with us. I cannot wait to have you home to meet your brother and the entire family. Your grandparents, aunts, uncles, and cousins are waiting to meet you. They send all their love."

"My beautiful daughter. I love you with all my soul and am proud of you. You are a strong and impressive warrior. You always amaze me. I have loved you since I knew you were in my belly. Every day, I love you more and more. I will be with you always. I Love you!"

"While writing this letter, the doctors told me your surgery was successful! I love you, mama. Soon I will see you. Thank you, God."

I updated everyone who followed our daughter's journal and who prayed for her about her successful surgery.

Following the surgery, she recovered quickly. She smiled and appeared happier than before the surgery. This procedure changed her and our lives.

That day, the mother who helped and taught me to speak for my daughter visited me at the hospital, and because of COVID-19, we had to meet outside. She brought presents for my son and daughter and food for me. I told her she was our angel who saved our daughter's life. Our girl was saved because of her knowledge of achondroplasia, kindness, and caring ways. Thank you.

Doctors did expect the decompression surgery to help with her central apnea, but we had to wait a few days before doing a sleep study to see the comparison. We discovered her central apnea had improved, so it was no longer a concern. Time would tell

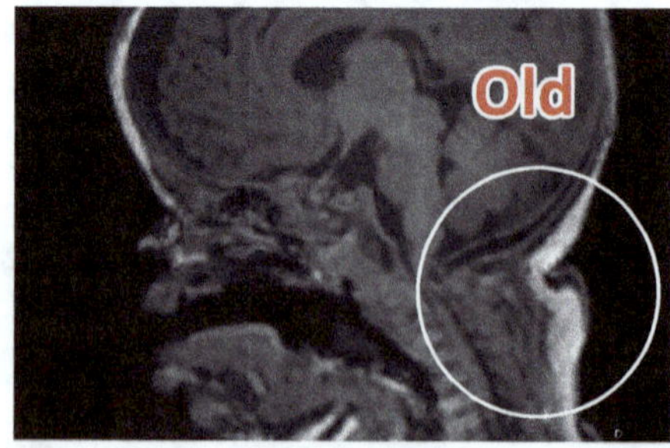

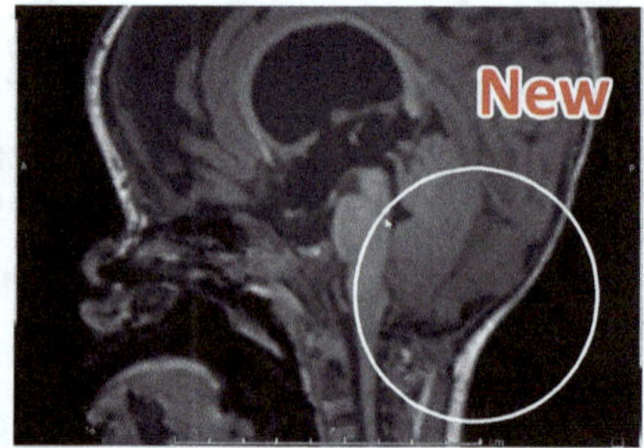

if the severe obstructive apnea would adjust to the new changes.

As the days passed, she did not need help to wake up or catch her breath to raise her oxygen levels. While feeding and burping, her oxygen levels remained normal. Relief and excitement replaced the heavy weight on my chest. I was so thankful.

The Children's Hospital of Westmead, Sydney, recommends that when burping your baby, hold them upright against your chest, with extra support on the head, neck, and back, and firmly rub their back. Their back is supported better than when placing the infant on your lap to burp.

A few days later, we started physical therapy. The therapist wanted to practice sitting her up to help strengthen her muscles, thus placing her in a "C" position. I remembered reading about this on the Moms Group and other achondroplasia groups. That we must prevent any sitting "C" positions to prevent complications.

I asked the physical therapist not to place her in a sitting position and explained why I did not want her to do this. She seemed upset because she had been an experienced therapist for over eleven years However, she had never treat an infant with achondroplasia. She agreed to wait for more information.

I signed on to the groups and asked them if placing an

achondroplasia infant in a sitting position was okay. A mom who has achondroplasia contacted me.

"Please do not let the therapist sit or practice sitting positions with your daughter," she pleaded. "I will drive to the hospital with copies of *Achondroplasia Pediatrics.* Give a copy to the therapist."

The kindness and helpful information from everyone I had spoken to about us was daunting. This woman drove one hour to the hospital to meet with me. Not only did she bring several copies of Achondroplasia Pediatrics, but she also brought food and presents. We had a wonderful time talking and learning about each other.

It is my first meeting with a person with achondroplasia. She was beautiful, intelligent, and kind. She showed me how incredible our daughter's life could be; it was a blessing to meet her. I gave the therapist a copy of Achondroplasia Pediatrics. We placed a copy in our daughter's room and gave another copy to the team of doctors.

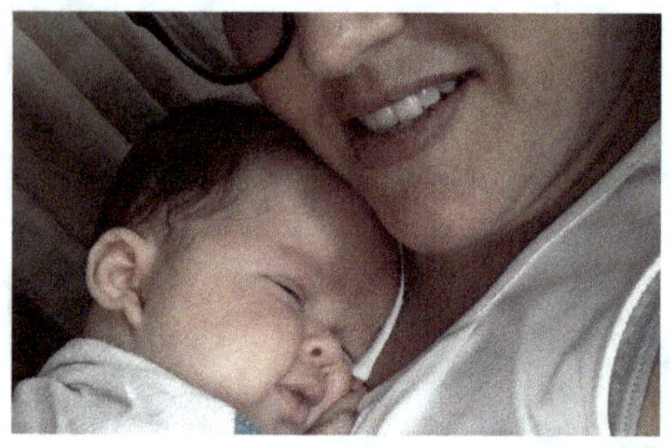

September 22 was a day to celebrate! Our daughter turned two months old and celebrated her first day without oxygen. Finally, I could see her beautiful face, clean of tape and tubes.

The Sleep Technologist performed a night sleep study, or polysomnography, on September 24th. The technician said that doing a sleep study during regular sleep hours would have more accuracy.

While visiting our daughter one weekend, a neurosurgeon I had never met came into the room to check on her. He said she needed an emergency CAT or CT scan because it looked like she had hydrocephalus, which occurs when fluid builds up in the skull and causes brain swelling.

"She will need surgery to place a shunt to drain the fluids," he said. "I am sure your doctors will agree with me.

I was in shock, and my emotions threatened to overwhelm me. It is like she had all the possible complications a child with achondroplasia can get. I walked around and tried to calm myself with deep breathing and praying. I started asking questions and researching.

Talk with your geneticist about an achondroplasia head circumference growth chart. The growth chart shows the average growth in babies with achondroplasia. Follow these steps to measure your child's head circumference.

1.- Wrap a flexible, non-stretchable measuring tape around their head at the widest part. This will be just above the eyebrows and ears and around the back, where the head slopes up prominently from the neck.

2.- Measure your baby's head at the spot with the largest circumference.

3.- Take the measurement three times and choose the largest size to the nearest 0.1 cm.

If your child experiences any of the following symptoms, they may need an evaluation from a neurosurgeon for hydrocephalus: headaches, irritability, lethargy, bulging fontanelle, sunsetting of the eye, and vomiting.

I asked her neurosurgeon to check the images and seek a neurosurgeon from the Little People of America Medical Board for their opinion. Both surgeons reviewed the images and agreed that she did not need a shunt.

Our daughter was getting better daily, and the medical team was preparing for us to go home. Her central apnea was under control, and she was resolving her obstructive apnea independently.

She did not need help to raise her oxygen levels. Doctors hoped her apnea would improve as she grew and gained muscle strength.

While in the hospital, I contacted a genetic doctor who specializes in achondroplasia. Two of my friends, one with achondroplasia, and the other has a son with hypo-achondroplasia, recommended her. I wanted this doctor to care for my daughter.

The doctor called me to check on my daughter's care. She carefully review my daughter's chart and explained about achondroplasia, the care needed, precautions to watch for, and follow-ups.

She continually checked her chart and updated me on her progress. She was there for us.

It is essential to request a car seat test before going home. The test takes about forty-five minutes to two hours. During testing, the examiner will monitor the baby's oxygen levels.

Because of her apnea and kyphosis, we bought a car seat bed in case she failed the regular car seat test. We placed her in the infant car seat on her car test day. She squirmed uncomfortably in the sitting position, and her oxygen levels dropped. She failed the test.

We then placed her on the car seat bed, and she passed the

car seat bed test. A specialist for car seat beds helped me with proper installation.

We were almost ready to go home.

To go home, she would need a follow-up pediatrician appointment three to five days after her release from the hospital. I called a pediatrician to schedule an appointment. We had spoken many times, and he agreed to see her and learn about her condition.

We had to reschedule twice with the pediatrician because she was not ready to leave the hospital.

Finally, when the doctors said she could go home, I called to schedule her follow-up appointment. The nurse told me the pediatrician decided that he could not take her on as a patient.

Because of her health issues, he felt that she needed another pediatrician that had experience in caring for achondroplasia. Therefore we had to stay at the hospital for two more days until I located another pediatrician. After many calls to doctors' offices and the insurance carrier, we found a pediatrician who is willing to take her and scheduled the follow-up appointment. We were now ready to go home.

It was October 2nd when the hospital discharged my daughter. Our son met his sister for the first time. "She is so cute," he said. He wanted to hug and kiss her. Her weight was 10.26 lbs., And she was 20.47 inches long.

My mother, son, daughter, and I left the hospital too late to avoid traffic, so the two-hour drive home became a four-hour nightmare. Traffic was heavy, and I had to feed her every three hours. It was dark outside when I pulled over on the freeway to feed her. I brought my daughter to the front seat with me and tried to put her into a position that protect her back while giving her the bottle.

The drive tired my son, so he climbed on my back, wanting attention and hugs. (The pulse oximeter machine started beeping because the oxygen went down). I got into the back seat with my son, a car seat, and a car seat bed, holding my daughter to troubleshoot the machine. The beeping sound from the machine frightened him because he feared something bad would happen to his baby sister.

There was no room to sit, so I squatted on the car floor.

My poor mother felt terrible because she could not help. She slid into the driver's seat and drove us home.

Suddenly, the oximeter machine turned off. I wanted to cry because I was so scared and thought, what more could go wrong?

Finally, we arrived home. My dad and husband already waited outside the house. This was the first time my dad saw his newborn granddaughter, and it was only the second time my husband held her. He hugged and kissed her, while saying, "How beautiful and precious she is."

I charged the battery but could not get the pulse oximeter machine to work even after charging. At midnight, a replacement pulse oximeter arrived. I discovered that the battery lasts only two hours.

It was our first night home, and her oxygen level dropped to 64 often. My heart told me to take her back to the hospital because she had not cry or wake up to eat. I had to wake her up periodically to feed her. Was it the machine causing the oxygen level discrepancies? or Was she having more health problems?

Our daughter was an active, two-month-old baby when we left the hospital. Now, she become weak, like when she was a newborn.

Watching her go through this frightened us.

"She is suffering," my husband said. "She is having trouble breathing."

My husband and I returned with her to the children's hospital emergency room, leaving our son with our family. Our daughter was having trouble with oxygen circulation.

With obstructive sleep apnea (OSA), the obstruction

She was not adequately expelling air; she was holding oxygen in. The hospital re-admitted her.

She had another sleep study performed at night. We tried different machines to see which worked better on her sleep apnea: CPAP and BiPAP machines (*Dubs, 2023*).

An ENT recommended a tracheostomy, an opening in the windpipe made to relieve an obstruction to breathing.

While figuring out what would work for her, the doctors performed a laryngoscopy on her narrow airway using an i-scoop procedure (*Raymondos, 2015*). My daughter did not need a tracheostomy.

Because she needed higher pressure for her treatment, the pulmonologist recommended the BiPAP. Our new routine was to teach her to sleep six to eight hours through the night so we would not have to remove the face mask. She would get her food nutrients and release her energy during the day. Our stay in the

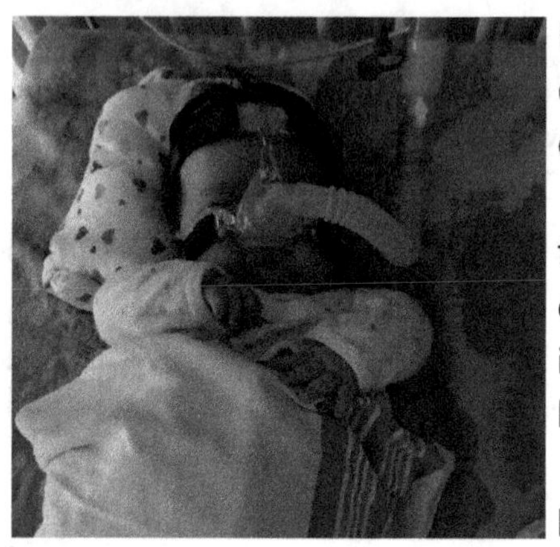

NICU was nineteen days, and during that time, I learned to operate the BiPAP machine.

Teaching her to wear a facial breathing mask was not easy. I looked for ways to trick her into wearing the breathing mask, like when she was sleeping.

One day, while I was in the bathroom, a new nurse training to care for her came into the room. My daughter was awake, so the nurse tried to place the mask on her face. I rushed out of the bathroom when I heard my baby screaming.

"Please stop and take the mask off her face!" I said to the nurse. "You are scaring her!"

"You have to get used to this," she said. "This is her new life."

That cruel statement upset me. "Just because she needs a machine does not mean she has to suffer!" I replied.

The nurse recognized her cruel words and apologized.

We can make medical procedures easier for our children with patience and understanding.

While in the NICU, I researched better cribs for her. I wanted a crib that would be difficult for my toddler son to enter. But I wanted easy access to take my daughter in and out and protect her back while putting her in the crib.

I found a beautiful crib where the side door opened, making it easy to reach in and get my baby. The family who presented it felt we were the best match. Their son had the opposite diagnosis from our daughter. He had Marfan syndrome (Mayo Clinic), a connective tissue disorder that affects the heart, eyes, blood vessels, and skeleton.

I connected with this mother because she was in my position over twenty-three years ago. Then, there was no Facebook or the Internet like today.

"It was hard," she said, "to find information about my son's diagnosis of Marfan syndrome."

Persons with Marfan syndrome are unusually tall and have spindly arms, legs, fingers, and toes. Because this syndrome affects the entire body, they are at risk for various complications, most notably cardiovascular complications.

Like our daughter, her son's diagnosis was uncommon. It is heartbreaking and lonely when you do not know where to seek help. Since then, more ways exist to research and connect with others for medical information.

God kept sending angels. Thank you.

Finally, my baby was ready to leave the children's hospital. We went home with a pulse oximeter, BiPAP machine, and a home health nurse follow-up the next day.

The insurance approved an appointment with a Bridge Clinic. A Bridge Clinic is an outpatient clinic that helps parents transition from NICU to home. After only three months of life, our daughter was ready to go home and stay home. Welcome home, beautiful girl! We are now complete!

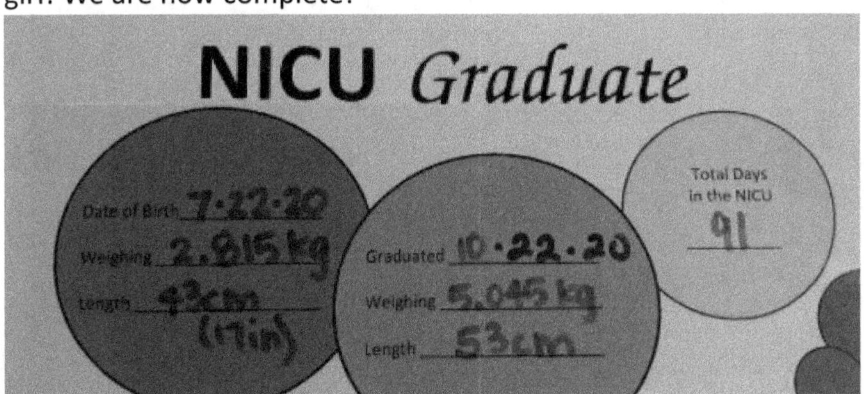

Part Six
Home

Support for our family continued to grow, and I thanked God for sending me extra angel eyes. A home health nurse arrived the following morning after our discharge from the children's hospital. She helped our transition from NICU to home and ensured our daughter had everything she needed in case of emergency.

"My job here is to prevent rehospitalization," she said.

The nurse had many years of nursing experience. She knew how to set up a house for good home care but had no experience with achondroplasia, but she was willing to learn. So, I assembled a folder with achondroplasia information and appropriate care for her.

She gave us emergency numbers and asked that we call with any questions, no matter the time of day. She also made sure the equipment functioned well. Together, we set up a schedule for follow-up appointments with the Bridge Clinic, pulmonologist, neurosurgeon, gastroenterologist, and primary doctor.

If you are familiar with the pulse oximeter, you will know that false alarms happen constantly. It is a nightmare! I was thankful for the machine and fine with waking up to false alarm.

I learned to read our daughter and knew if she was in distress. I learned to listen to the machine's alarms. When the machine beeped twice and stopped, I knew she was okay.

The pulse oximeter was like a mechanical angel checking her. I am thankful that I have not had to awaken her from an apneic episode.

After arriving home, I reorganized the room we shared. I made a corner where our son could have space with his toys and books.

I did not want him to notice a significant change in the family dynamics. He was now a big brother, curious about his new sister, and had many questions.

"She is so cute, mama. I want to hug and squeeze her, but I am scared I might hurt her," he said. "Why is she wearing a giraffe mask on her face?" He asked about the BiPAP mask with the long hose connected to the breathing machine.

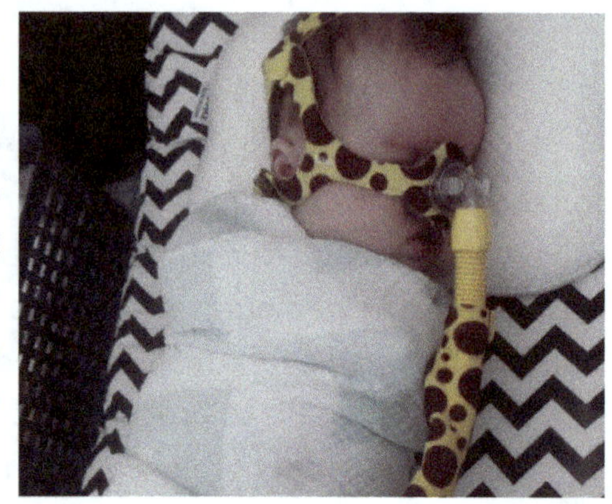

I placed our daughter's crib in another corner next to our bed. I wanted her to feel safe and next to me so I could closely watch her. The crib was perfect, and the mattress was firm enough to protect her back. This worked wonderfully for tummy time.

Tummy time is good for newborns to help them develop neck control and strengthen their muscles to roll over, sit up, crawl, and walk. This helps strengthen their muscles, allowing them to crawl, walk, roll over, and sit independently. This is especially important for babies with achondroplasia who may develop complications because of spinal kyphosis.

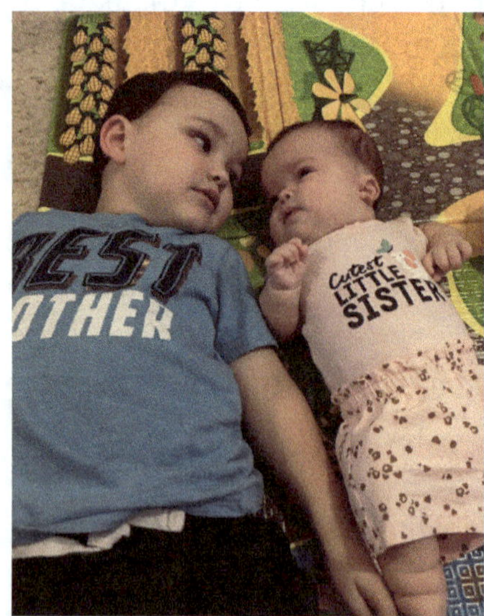

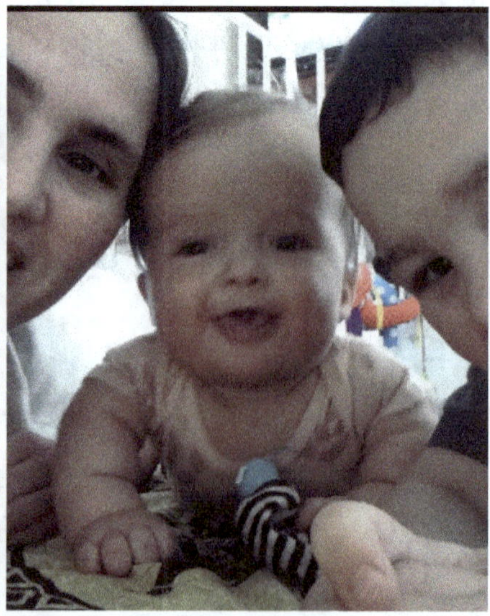

Tummy time is so-called by placing your baby's belly down on your chest. You may also place the infant on a firm surface like a floor or crib with a firm mattress.

Always stay with your baby during this time. Never leave your baby alone during tummy time, especially if your baby cannot control their head or roll over independently. Place your baby on their back, never their belly, when they are ready to sleep. This helps to prevent sudden infant death syndrome (SIDS).

We wanted to keep our daughter happy, healthy, and out of the hospital. She was high-risk and needed twenty-four-hour attention. She could quickly get sick because of her small airway, apnea, and the pandemic from coronavirus. A baby with achondroplasia has a small airways and lung spaces and can develop complications, even with a simple cold.

Because of her obstructive sleep apnea, her risk of SIDS were higher.

Before her birth and I knew about her achondroplasia diagnosis, and I bought everything a baby needed. I bought a car seat, bathtub, and feeding chair; everything I loved when our son was a baby. After her birth, I discovered none of the items suited her unique needs.

In addition to the car seat bed that helped to keep her airway open and her spine straight, we purchased other items unique to her needs. The feeding chair was at a 45-degree angle in a sitting position until she could do it independently. The bathtub needed to be longer so I could keep her back straight and her head and neck in a neutral plane aligned with the spine to facilitate breathing. A bassinet stroller works as a bed and chair with a stiff back.

I discovered our daughter qualified for disability, which allowed me to stay home and have a part-time nurse to help with her care. The nurse caring for her allowed me to spend quality time with our toddler son and time for myself, allowing me to schedule follow-up appointments.

Once I read that a sibling of a sibling with disabilities can feel invisible. Is what they call it "a glass child" (Parents.com). After knowing that, I wanted to make sure my son didn't feel invisible so I gave him additional care too.

Our son saw his sister connected to the machines. Having a sibling with a medical condition is difficult, especially when you are three years old and do not understand what is happening. It was hard to see him struggling because something could happen to his baby sister. He would ask, "What happens if she stops breathing? Can she die?"

He had heard the noises coming from the devices and knew it meant something big when we rushed to his sister's side when the alarms went off. He was curious about her health and why she needed the machine.

He learned the meanings of the flashing red warning light and the steady green light and alerted us when he heard the alarm. He soon learned not to worry when the machine beeped. He would run to check on her and say, "Mommy, she is okay; I can see her breathing."

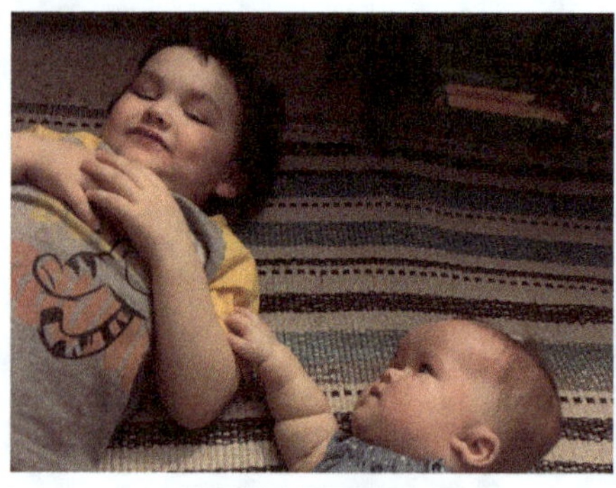
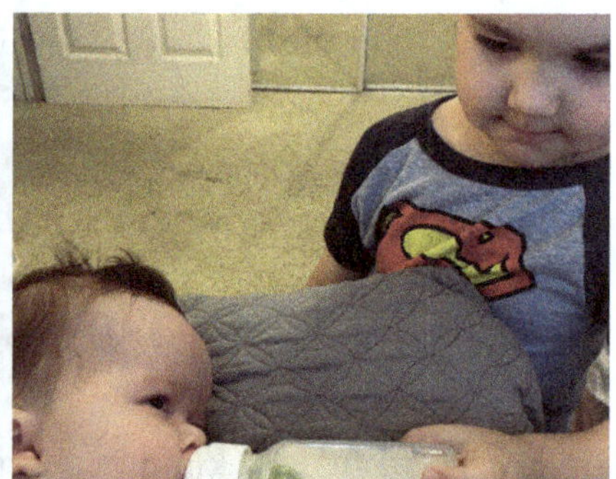
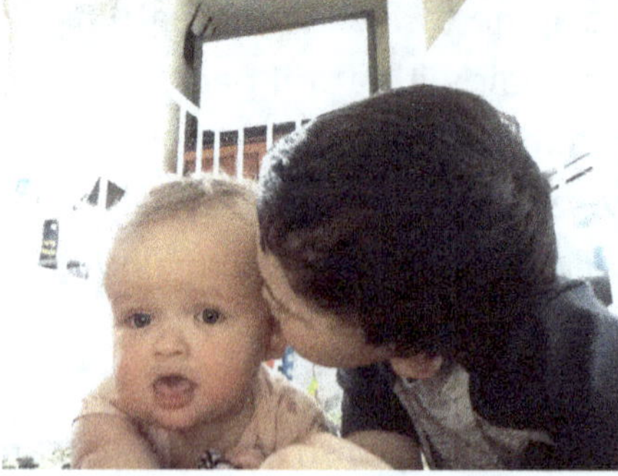
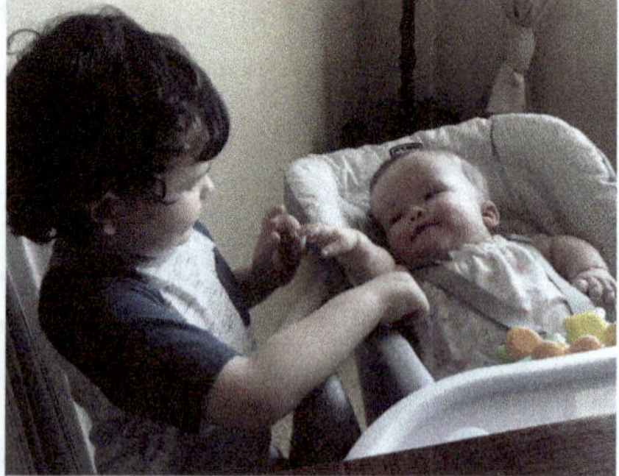

Our son and I worried about her, but this time together allowed us to discuss our feelings and collect our thoughts. When he and I interacted, I realized how mature this three-year-old had become since his sister's arrival. We knew this was a difficult time for our son so we gave him extra attention. We included him in all her care and explained what we were doing and why.

Watching our toddler, I noticed his empathy toward others, especially those with obvious medical conditions or impairments, and what a wonderful human being he was becoming. Learning to view life in this different and beautiful way was something most children his age would not ever experience.

Until then, I had not realized the stress my body had gone through while carrying five extra weeks of amniotic fluid in my last trimester. The weight of the excess amniotic fluid was pushing my organs down and weighing heavy on my belly. I tired quickly, my back ached, and anxiety overwhelmed me because of the unknown and the pressure of learning to fight for our daughter's life. I suffered from infections, causing mastitis and pain from the c-section stitches and mastitis. I had ignored my body talking to me, so I would put on stress-weight and had no energy.

Mentally, it took time to erase the NICU mode of unpleasant feelings that left a mark on my heart and mind. In the NICU, alarms were constantly going off, machines were beeping, and medical staff came in and out hourly. I felt guilt and blame because I could not breastfed her as I did with our son. I could not hold or bond with her in this beautiful way. Watching other parents go through the same experience was stressful, sad, and heartbreaking.

Like most mothers, we prepared a nursery and looked forward to waking up with our family to start the day in the comfort of our home. It is a hard feeling to explain, but it changes you as a person when you live life in a NICU. A NICU parent can understand those feelings. It is essential to rest and not forget about your health because our kids need us to be strong, healthy, and we want to be there for them.

I had dreamed of having many children. I struggled with many issues in my little family. Dealing with another pregnancy would have been difficult. My husband wrestled with depression, which became worse when COVID-19 hit. Our daughter had many medical issues and possible surgeries. Our son worried about us.

I decided to tie my tubes and did not regret my decision. It was not an easy decision because I feared the surgical risks, but I could now concentrate on our children and marriage. I could not ask for anything more.

Our daughter's insurance approved her for a program that helped with early intervention in developmentally delayed children. The program met once a week online because COVID-19 would not let us meet in person, and it covered all her milestones.

Our instructor did not know about achondroplasia but was ready and willing to learn.

Shortly after arriving home, our daughter developed scaly skin and a rash over her face and body. We did not know what it was. Was it her new environment? Is it from changing her formula from liquid to powder?

The dermatologist recommended corticosteroids and antibacterial creams. The creams had an adverse effect and caused hives. After speaking with her doctor, we stopped the creams to consult with a pediatric dermatologist.

We knew it was eczema (*Mayo Clinic*), but no medications were helping. Her skin looked like it was getting worse.

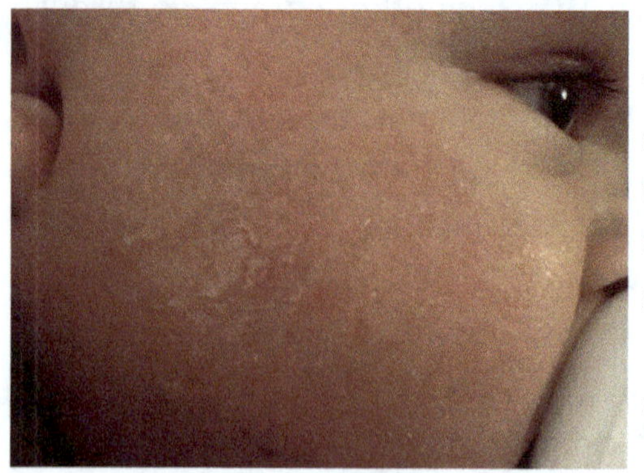

A rash covered her face and spread everywhere, including the folds of her skin, so when she scratched, her skin broke open and bled.

While researching what was happening with

her skin, we discovered the exact cause of eczema was unknown, but, it was associated with an overactive immune system response. Her doctor ordered allergy tests for fear that allergies could cause swelling of her small airway. We treated eczema with an elimination diet until our pediatric dermatologist appointment.

With the allergist, we discovered that she had allergies to eggs, milk, turkey, chicken, oats, wheat, dogs, and cats. We found that soy and almonds triggered her eczema. Knowing that helped me to help her with her eczema.

Finally, we had our appointment with the pediatric dermatologist, but that treatment did not work either.

A childhood friend of mine helped us with our daughter's eczema and topical steroid withdrawal (TSW). We placed her on a clean diet to cleanse the steroid cream from her body.

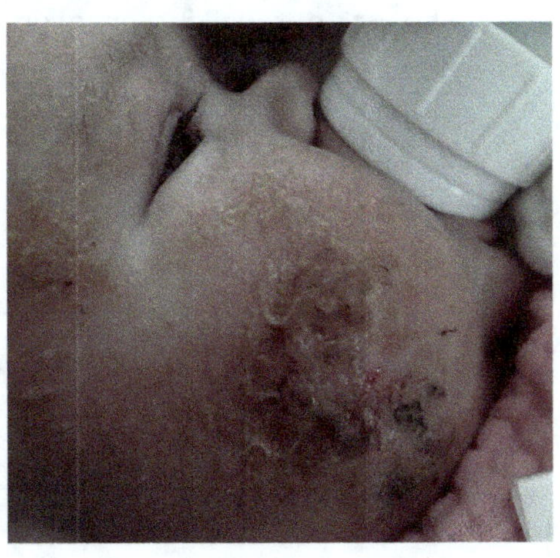

It was not easy watching her beautiful face go through the ravages of a reaction to the cream and then through withdrawal. However, her skin was healthy and healing beautifully after a few months. She still had eczema patches, but her skin did not bleed when scratched.

The eczema was an overwhelming experience for us. I was thankful for my friend's guidance and emotional support because this would not have been easy without her.

Good nutrition is good practice for GERD, eczema, and obesity. In achondroplasia, the potential for obesity is high. Obesity will affect the spine and legs, causing bowed legs and placing pressure on the spine that can lead to pain.

The neurosurgeon ordered an MRI to check her decompression surgery progress and for signs of hydrocephalus.

She never showed signs of hydrocephalus; we took precautions and measured her head, but we measured three times to ensure we had the correct measurement. The doctor asked that we measure more often and may have to do something if the head circumference reaches fifty. Because of our daily measurement routine, the doctor discovered a difference.

While driving home from our MRI appointment, the neurosurgeon called and told us she was developing hydrocephalus. The MRI results showed there was fluid buildup in her brain.

"The extra fluids on her brain are pushing her head out," the doctor said. "I am concerned this may affect her neurological development and speaking ability and mobility."

She was not walking or talking yet, so it was hard to know if hydrocephalus affected these areas. While in the NICU, she was not repositioned from side to side, so her head was slightly flat on one side. We talked about a helmet but decided against it.

We discussed an ETV, Endoscopic Third Ventriculostomy (*Memorial et al. Center*).

An ETV is an alternative procedure to shunt surgery.

Instead of inserting a shunt, the surgeon makes a hole in the third ventricle floor of the brain where the cerebral spinal fluid drains and the body absorbs it.

Located and stored in the ventricle cavities of the brain is a protective fluid called cerebral spinal fluid. The ventricles swell if the cerebral spinal fluid cannot drain. The swelling ventricles put pressure on the brain and skull and cause an enlarged.

We scheduled an ETV surgical procedure for the next available day.

After hanging up the phone from the doctor, I could not speak. Have you ever felt like you froze after receiving bad news? That was precisely how I felt, frozen. I had no words and no expression. It was like I could not believe what I had just heard, but at the same time, it did not surprise me. All we could do was keep believing and moving forward.

On May 4th, my husband, our eight-month-old daughter, and I returned to the children's hospital for an ETV five days after the MRI.

My husband and I waited in the waiting room. Finally, we saw on the screen that her surgeon had completed the surgery. The neurosurgeon talked to us and let us know that everything went well.

"Cleaning her eczema before the surgery took extra time, but everything went smoothly. I did not see any damage to her brain,

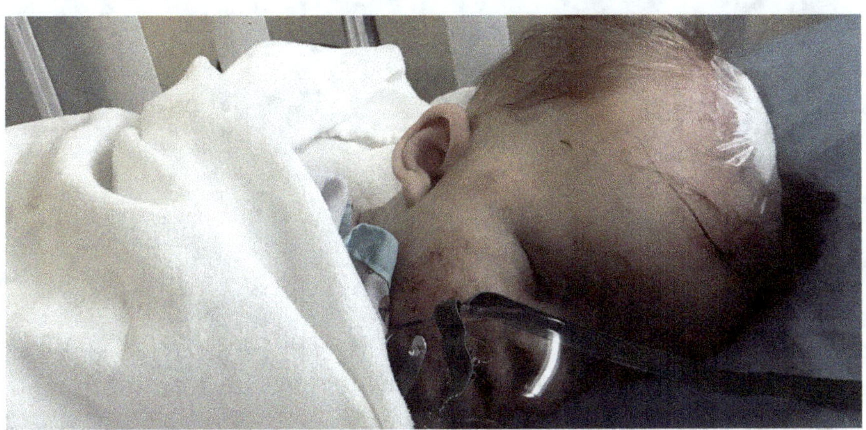

which is good," he said. "With the ETV, insure that she is at an upright angle to help the ETV drain the cerebral spinal fluid."

When she woke up from surgery, she cried and screamed. She had not eaten for many hours, so I knew she was hungry and possibly hurting from the surgical pain.

Seeing her cry like this was abnormal because she was an easy, sweet baby. Her screams broke our hearts.

My husband teared up, listening to her screams, helpless to ease her pain. From that day on, she feared people who looked like doctors and seemed upset at me for letting this happen to her.

We fed her and gave her pain medication. Soon after, she fell asleep. When she awoke, it was like nothing had happened; she was happy and smiling. She was unbelievably strong, and once home, we noticed the improvement. She started making more progress with mobility. It was like she had never had surgery. She laughed and rolled around with her brother.

Our daughter was doing great. After four months of staying home, she was finally strong and healthy enough to leave the house to visit our extended family. It took some preparation to gather all

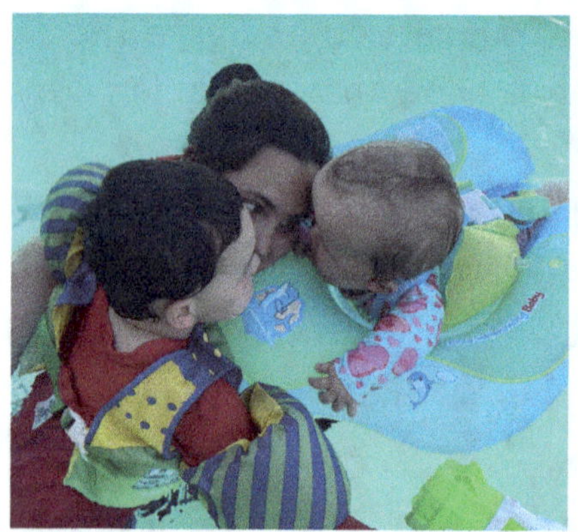
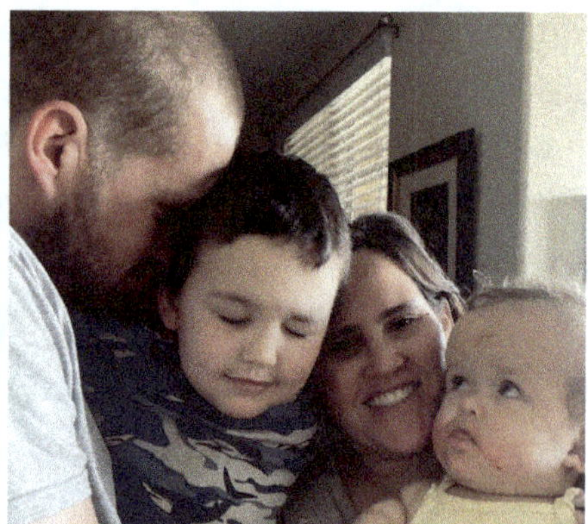

the items she would need before we left our home. We spent more time loading the car than we did at our destination.

Our family fell in love with her but feared they might hurt her. It took some time for them to feel comfortable enough to carry her. During this gathering, my dad proudly held her for the first time.

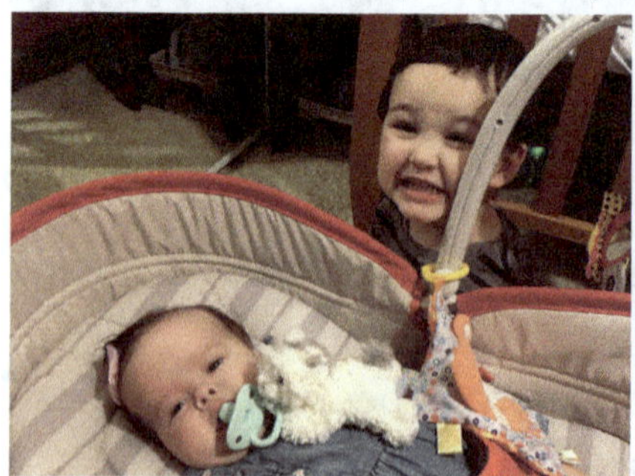
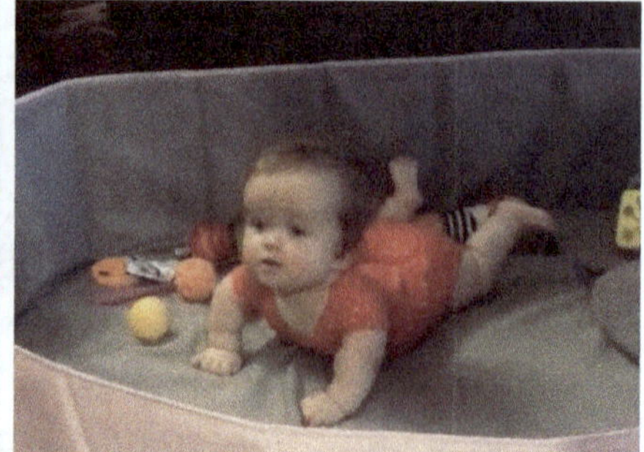

We had fun interacting with our daughter and son simultaneously. Her health was improving, and when the Sleep Technician performed another sleep study, it showed that her obstructive apnea had improved from severe to moderate.

I was bathing her at night on June 18, 2021. She loved bath time, and while gently drying her head, I saw a drop of fluid on her stitches. Frightened but calm, I saw her last stitch coming out, so I asked my dad for a magnifying glass. I made a video and sent it to her neurosurgeon, a good doctor who always responded to my questions.

He immediately returned my email and told me he was out of the city. "You can wait for me to return on Monday," he said, "or another doctor from my team can help you at my office."

I chose to go to his office the next day, Friday. I drove to the children's hospital with my mom, daughter, and son, hoping the doctor would say everything would be okay.

Sadly, the appointment did not go as how I thought; when they touched the incision they saw more fluids coming out, so they sent her to the ER for a CT scan.

When the doctor came in, he said, "She has to stay in the hospital because she needs a shunt placement (*Johns Hopkins*)."

It frightened me because it was easy to confuse hydrocephalus in babies with achondroplasia. I did not want the shunt if there were alternatives.

The surgeon then explained, "We do not have any more choices. If we wait, there will be a risk of infection, which may lead to meningitis, hospitalization, and more complications. We can surgically check the ETV and see if it is draining. But then, we will need another surgery to place the shunt if the ETV is not working. Her fontanel may still be open, which could be why the fluid finds a way out."

"Or," he continued, "we go for one surgery and fewer complications by placing an adult shunt because her head is big enough. This prevents another surgery from replacing a shunt from infant to adult. This shunt has a programmable valve that we can non-surgically adjust." He added, "If she were my daughter, that is the alternative I would take."

I called the geneticist and asked her to speak with this doctor. She agreed with this doctor's assessment, so we went for the shunt placement. They admitted her to the hospital, and my mom and son drove home.

The following day, she had surgery. I fell apart while in the waiting room when my sister called. When I heard her voice, I could no longer control my emotions.

Through sobs, I told her I was not expecting another surgery. I was not ready for this and was not looking forward to spending time in the NICU again, going through that emotional roller coaster.

"These last eight months, I watched my daughter's health improve," I said. "The NICU feelings finally left, but now it may happen again."

Despite my worries, the surgery went well, and she woke up happy and hungry. We are back home. We can see the shunt is working, and we do not have to worry about positioning her at an angle to help the extra fluids drain, as we did with the ETV. The shunt drain regardless of the position.

The early intervention specialist and I connected with a physical therapist from ALPE, an organization in Spain specializing in achondroplasia. Our first lesson was about gross-motor activities, large muscle groups of the human body that help with sitting, walking, and balancing.

Our main concern was kyphosis and placing our daughter in a sitting position. The Spanish therapist explained that sitting an achondroplasia infant up is not good when they are not ready to do so independently.

"When their bodies become strong," she said, "place them on your legs with their backs leaning on your chest, inclined. Sit them on the floor with you as back support for two minutes when their muscles strengthen. If they can hold their body up, do this twice daily but always have you as back support."

Many geneticists and adults with dwarfism do not recommend physical therapy because of the therapist's lack of knowledge about achondroplasia. However, physical therapists have other ways to help with activities, such as an exercise and stability ball to help balance.

COVID-19 infections were decreasing; businesses were opening and trying to return to everyday life. A friend told me that the Little People of America (LPA) decided to resume their meetings. One meeting was in my district. I contacted the LPA organization to subscribe, but eventually, we did not go because our daughter was a high-risk baby. Her geneticist recommended we do not attend and wait for COVID-19 cases to decrease.

An LPA member contacted us with the name of a family who lived nearby, and all have achondroplasia. This beautiful family came to visit us and meet our daughter. It is rewarding to meet people with the same diagnosis as your child and who are doing well in life. After meeting them, you forget about the diagnosis and only see amazing people talking with you, worrying about your daughter, and sharing their lives.

This family showed us all the fantastic things our daughter could do. They are professionals and own businesses; they are parents and children; they are great friends and caring people.

I am so thankful that God put them in our lives. Our daughter is teaching us many new things and opening doors to a beautiful world of diversity, kindness, and acceptance.

I spoke with our daughter's geneticist about physical therapy.

"Do not practice standing yet until she is about one year old," she said. "Her knee and ankle joints are loose, which is normal but should improve over time. She should start standing, holding onto something. Given her many hospitalizations and surgeries, she may need extra time to catch up."

The geneticist gave this information to the therapist:

1.- Use careful head and neck support, particularly with transitions.
2.- Prevent unsupported sitting or holding in a sitting position for too long until she can fully sit up and support her back independently.
3.- No swings or jumper seats that hang from doorways to prevent her from jumping around without head support.
4.- Use solid back strollers and other support. Do not use umbrella strollers that may forcibly flex the neck.
5.- Use a neck roll in strollers and car seats. When restrained, achondroplasia infants with large and prominent occiputs will have their necks in a forced flexed position. We want to avoid this. Ask your therapist to show you how to use the neck roll.

Our daughter's weekly early intervention class showed positive reports regarding her milestones. Her report showed she was a beginner in motor skills compared to babies without achondroplasia and babies with achondroplasia.

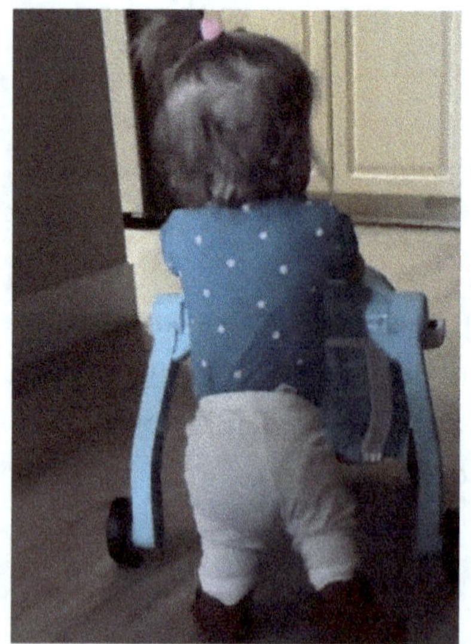

Babies with achondroplasia begin the course and catch up on their time and in their way, especially with the gross motor skills of the large muscle group like the arms and legs. Achondroplasia babies take more time to learn to walk and sit. Some babies learn to walk first. When their back muscles get strong, they learn to sit.

Today was a day to celebrate. Our daughter started pulling herself up and taking some steps. She looked happier, more confident, and able to do anything she wanted to do. I could not believe she was walking! Her independent, cheerful face was everything. She was eighteen months old, and her early intervention reports showed she was no longer behind.

She was behind on her motor skills because of her low muscle tone. Her low muscle tone kept her from performing motor skills milestones on time. Her time in the NICU and developing hydrocephalus did not help, but she finally mastered it. I was so proud of her because in what would have taken months to complete, she did in only one month.

An X-ray showed no issues with kyphosis during her orthopedic appointment.

Her geneticist recommended a hearing test every four months. She did not pass the hearing test in the first hospital, but she passed it after her decompression surgery.

We tried to have her BAER test (Krucik, 2017) done but could never finish the test because she was fussy and could not sleep for ninety minutes.

The doctor said she had some hearing loss and fluids in one ear. Because her small airway could lead to an infection and fluid in the internal ear canal could lead to hearing loss, the doctor transferred us to a new specialist for a sedated BAER test.

During the audiologist appointment, we discovered that she had fluid in one ear and wax buildup in the other ear. We had to resolve these issues before the sedated BAER test (brainstem auditory evoked response) could be performed.

People with achondroplasia have small canals in the external portion of their ear making it difficult to see deep inside to check for infections. It is essential to have an audiologist and ear, nose, and throat doctor (ENT). We had follow-up appointments with the ENT, a neurosurgeon, and a pulmonologist. Children with achondroplasia are prone to ear infections, fluid in the ear, and hearing loss.

We went to the ENT to check her ears. He cleaned the wax on one of her ears, confirmed fluids in the other, and recommended an ear tube.

Ear tube placement and tonsillectomy are standard procedures in babies with achondroplasia.

The ENT checked her tonsils and adenoids and recommended removal because they were too big for her airways and may cause her continued obstructive apnea. Her tongue was also more significant than when he last checked her.

It was our son's first year of school and a return to everyday life following COVID-19. However, a respiratory virus broke out shortly after starting school, infecting many children and teachers.

Our daughter was more fragile than her brother, so we had to take extra precautions. She became ill with rhinovirus. Because of her sensitive immune system, she developed pneumonia and needed a five-day hospitalization, oxygen, and then oxygen support for seven more days at home.

She would have another MRI to check her decompression surgery and shunt function. The doctors scheduled her for tonsillectomy, adenoidectomy, and an ear tube placement.

Our daughter's follow-up sedated MRI showed that her shunt was over-draining. This was a concern because it showed she might need another brain surgery to replace the shunt. But, her doctor recommended waiting and monitoring her shunt's progress.

The MRI showed that she had an ear infection in both ears.

Two days before Christmas, she had surgery to place ear tubes and to shave and remove tonsils and adenoids. In the process, they discovered an even bigger ear infection.

Recovering from this last surgery was difficult. Thinking she would have pain scared me, but her bravery and strength amazed

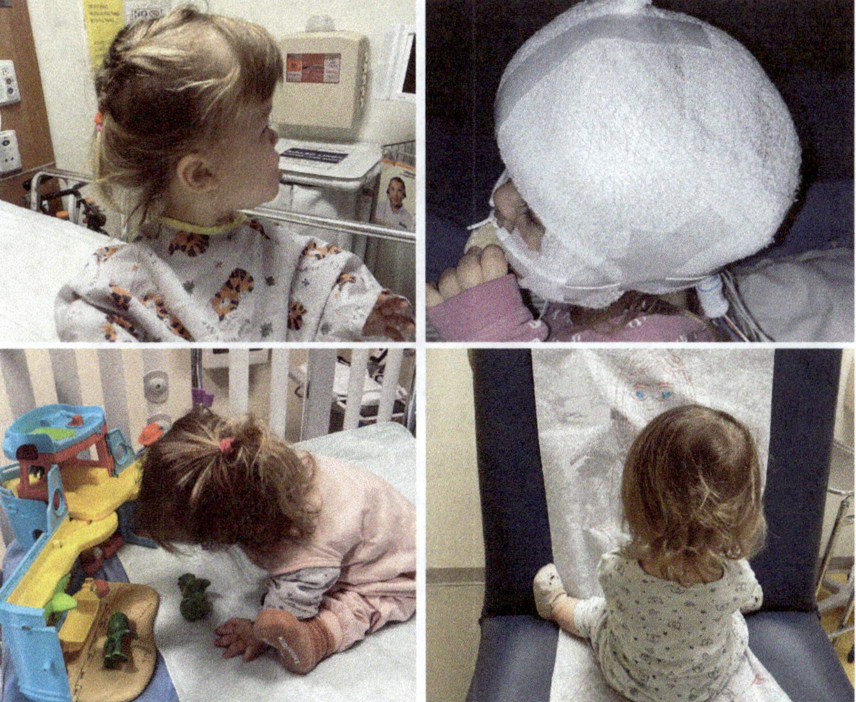

us. She had her sedated BAER test, which showed mild hearing loss.

The first two years of life for many babies with achondroplasia can be challenging: many doctors and appointments, and more and more surgeries similar to our daughter. Still, all babies with achondroplasia must need baseline tests to prevent complications before they get worse.

Knowing this, it was hard for my husband to think about the pregnancy, delivery, and our daughter's surgeries. When he did open up to others, he felt ill at ease that it might be information overload. However, he spent as much time as possible with our children.

He would play Star Wars with our son, swinging and jumping with their light sabers. Then, our daughter would grab her light saber and join the fight.

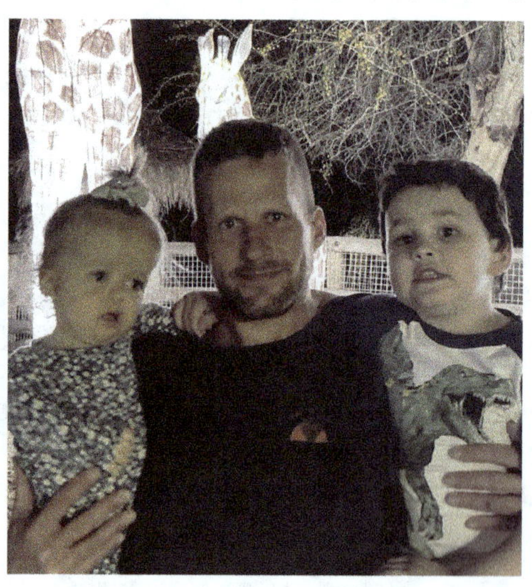

My daughter loved the Beatles, especially the uplifting ballad, *Hey Jude.* She and my husband would loudly sing this ballad, dance around, and scream like the Beatles' fans. Then, they would sit together, watch Mary Poppins, or dress up for a tea party.

My husband received so much enjoyment and loved every second he spent with her and our son.

I was amazed by how my son presented his sister to others and his understanding of her diagnosis. He now introduces his sister as his baby sister. "She is two, and I am five," he would say, "and she is really cute."

When he saw a surprised look on their faces or they

mentioned that she was small, he replied, "Yes, she has achondroplasia, and for that reason, she is smaller than other kids her age."

Our daughter is an incredible two-year-old girl who is happy, capable, loving, beautiful, dramatic, brave, and strong. She loves her brother and family, singing, counting, saying the ABCs, drawing, and having tea parties. She loves to look at playbooks, and her favorite treats are gummies.

I will not lie. Every procedure and every surgery she underwent was scary. I will say, however, that every surgery and procedure improved her life. I discovered, too, that every time something about her health frightened me, I knew there was a solution. I knew that everything would be okay.

Several months later, my daughter had another sleep study. The overjoyed doctor told us that she no longer needed the BiPap machine. Soon after, we had more wonderful news when our visit to the audiologist revealed that she no longer had hearing loss. From then on, we knew everything would be okay.

Epilogue

We had so much to be thankful for. Our two-year-old daughter was no longer afraid of going to her doctor's appointments. Instead, she would ask questions. "What are they going to do? Is it going to hurt? Can I help?"

One day, after seeing her doctor, we decided to turn our appointment days into a fun family outing. Even though we are not together we do everything possible to enjoy ourselves as a family. The day was sunny and warm; everyone was in good spirits, so we drove to the beach.

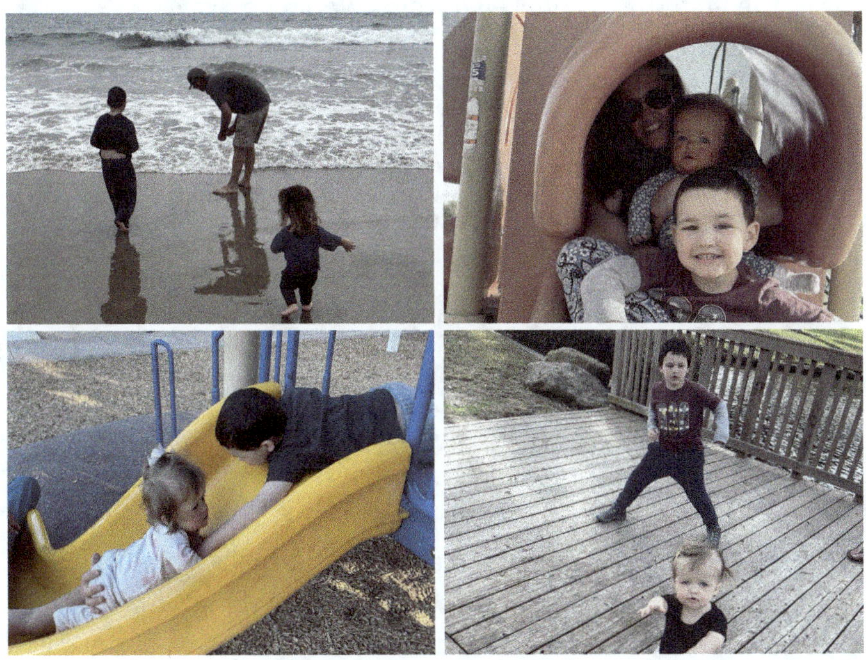

Watching our daughter and son frolicking together on the water's edge and running on the beach was terrific. We never thought we would see the day. Then, I told my husband everything would be okay.

When I am asked how I knew everything would be okay, I replied, "There were so many different and unique occasions when I prayed for everything to be okay. I looked forward to saying it every time we faced and overcame a hardship."

- When I first heard our baby cry, I knew everything would be okay.
- When we arrived at the new hospital, I knew everything would be okay.
- When she slept on my chest for the first time, and her peaceful, loving face faced mine, I knew everything would be okay.
- When God's presence saved me from depression, I knew everything would be okay.
- When she rolled over in bed and asked me for a hug for the first time, I knew everything would be okay.
- When she took her first steps, I knew everything would be okay.
- When our family and friends supported us, I knew every thing would be okay.
- Each time a surgical procedure went well, I knew everything would be okay.
- When we enjoyed our trips to our doctor's appointments because we made them family trips, I knew everything would be okay.
- When my son told me that his sister was the most beautiful girl in the world and that he loved her, I knew everything would be okay.
- When I watched my son and daughter play, dance, and pretend to be superheroes, I knew everything would be okay.
- When my children hugged each other every morning when they got out of bed, I knew everything would be okay.
- When my children lay in bed and spoke softly to each other, I knew everything would be okay.

Stay informed. One day, you will share this information with someone else and reach out to others, searching for answers.

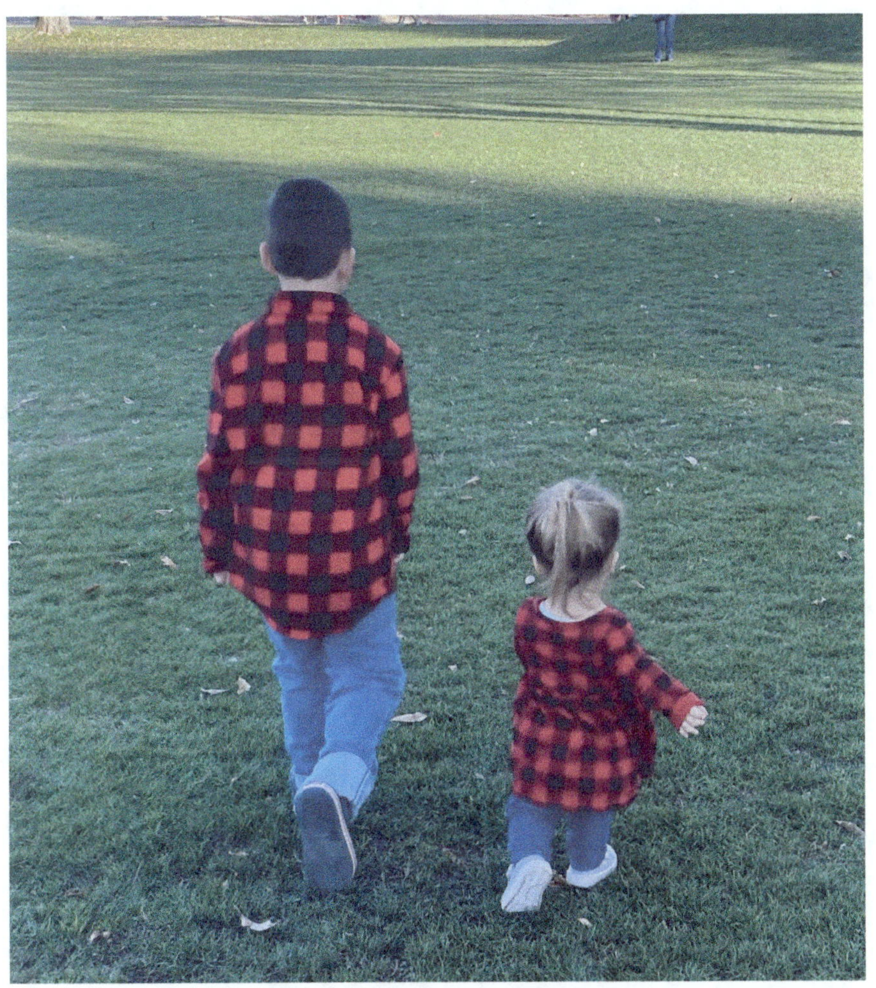

Everything will be okay.

Build your Medical Team

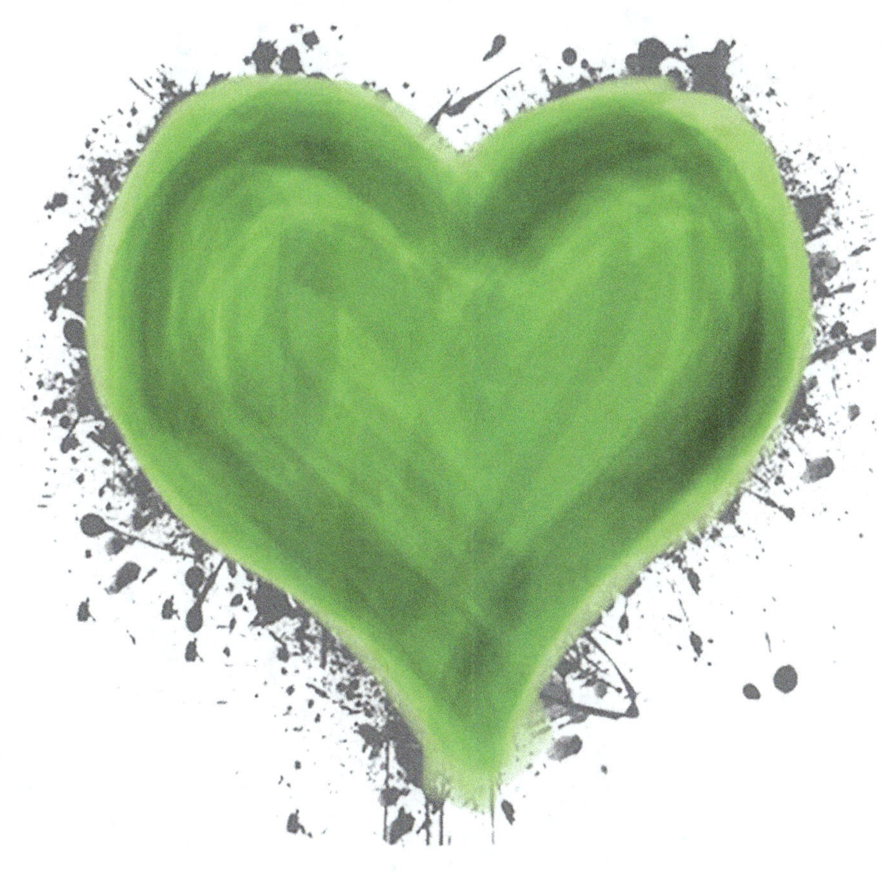

Get Ready, Be Prepared, Know the Signs

Your doctor has diagnosed your child with achondroplasia.
Take a deep breath because knowing the diagnosis is the first step
toward advocating for your child's care. Gather all the information
you can, enjoy the journey, and do not forget about yourself
because everything will be okay.

INFORMATION

Name:

____

Birthday:

____

Measurements:

____

Insurance:

____

____

____

Notes:

CARE RECOMMENDATIONS

Kyphosis (Page 41) (Page 63-64)

Children with achondroplasia may develop kyphosis. Also known as hunchback. Excessive upper back curvature. May cause pain and stiffness.

-A spinal XRay may be needed to check for kyphosis.

-Is crucial not to put a child with Achondroplasia in a sitting or "C" position until they are ready to sit on their own.

-Babies born with a spine curve, or kyphosis, get better when they walk on their own.

-Avoid unsupported sitting; place a child on their back on a hard surface, like the floor, to reduce or remove the kyphosis risk.

-No swings.

-No bouncers.

-No Umbrella stroller.

Tummy time (Page 52-53)

-Time spent by a baby lying on their stomach while awake.

-Helps with bonding and protects the back.

-Use a crib for tummy time.

-Use a Pack and Play bed.

-Use a water mat.

-Use a small plastic pool.

-Use the floor.

-This helps to keep the back straight.

Small Airways

Because of small airways and runny noses, keep these items at home.

a. Saline drops

b. Humidifier

c. Nasal aspirator

Pulse Oximeter

purshase one to monitor your baby's blood oxygen level while you wait for baseline testing. Ask your doctor for information on baby pulse oximeters. Baby pulse oximeters may be expensive and covered by insurance if prescribed by a doctor.

-Learn how to read the machines.
-Learn how to read your child.

Head Circunference (Page 43)

Purchase a soft tape measure to measure head circumference and a notebook to record results

-Add the date and time of day when recording.
-Measure once monthly but measure three times for accuracy.
-Notify the doctor if the measurement falls outside the normal range.
-Ask your doctor for the signs and symptoms of hydrocephalus.
-Ask your doctor for a head circumference chart for achondroplasia.

Gastroesophageal reflux disease (GERD) (Page 37)

-Common in babies with an achondroplasia diagnosis.
-Required medication.
-Causes heartburn and regurgitation.
- Can lead to breathing problems.

Anesthesia (Page 39)

-Risk are higher because small airways and tracheas.

-Dose should be related to weight.

-If require intubation be more careful because the small air ways

-Carefully support the head during and after the anesthesia since the head is more prominent and the neck smaller.

BUILD YOUR SUPPORT SYSTEM

Join research groups. Look for organizations familiar with achondroplasia, dwarfism, or dysplasia. Connect with others and learn about the diagnosis. Meet doctors and specialists and enjoy different activities, seminars, therapies, special events, and consultation. Meet other families and people with achondroplasia.

Groups I recommend:

-"Achondroplasia" Group on Facebook.

-"PLOP" Parents with child with Achondroplasia Group on Facebook.

-The Magic Foundation for Children's Growth (www.magic foundation.org).

-Little People of America and if you are in United State find your district of Little People of America

-ALPE of Spain specializes in achondroplasia and dysplasia's. You do not have to live in Spain or speak Spanish to join this group.

- Little Legs Big Heart Foundation

- MyAchonJourney.com

BABY ITEMS YOU WILL NEED

Car seat bed

-If your baby does not pass the car seat test.

-Keeps back straight and airways open.

-Recommended for the first few months.

Car seat

-Ask for a car seat test before going home.

-Look for a car seat with a flat, stiff, straight back.

-Do not get a car seat that pushes your infant's head for
ward. For example, the extent forever car seat.

-Because of their small airways and low muscle tone, do not
allow any baby to take long naps in the car seat, especially
those with achondroplasia.

-While respecting the car seat limit laws, the longer you can
keep your baby in the rear position before forward and for
ward position before the booster, the better for the child.

Stroller

-Look for a stroller with good back support.

-A bassinet stroller works best. The stroller can be
repositioned to a high chair. This helps when starting solid
foods.

-No umbrella strollers.

Infant bathtub

-Look for one that is firm and will keep the back straight.

-Aligns the spine.

-Has an incline to keep airways open.

-A long bin with a large sponge to support the body worked
best.

High chair

-Flat and straight back for good spine control.

-Reclining high chair because it will start eating at a forty-five-degree angle.

- You can use a bassinet stroller as a high chair.

Medical items that can help you at home.

a. Pulse Oximeter

b. Thermometer

c. Stethoscope

d. Infant blood pressure monitor

e. Otoscope

Other recommended items:

Play items to help build motor skills. Set up a playroom where they can play and grow independently. These items engage curiosity, allow them to pull themselves up, help them climb, and help them hold themselves up.

a. Sensory toys.

b. Styrofoam stacking blocks.

c. Tricycle.

d. Pack and play.

e. Water floor mat.

f. Small activity table.

g. Mirrors.

h. Arts and crafts.

i. Self-discovery

MEDICAL INFORMATION

Build your Team of Doctors.Look for doctors that specialize in Achondroplasia or are willing to learn.

Pediatrician:

Name: ____

Phone: ____

Address: ____

____

Notes: ____

____

____

Genetics:

Name: ____

Phone: ____

Address: ____

____

Notes: ____

____

____

Neurosurgeon:

Name: ____

Phone: ____

Address: ____

____

Notes: ____

____

____

Pulmonologist:

Name: _______________________________________

Phone: _______________________________________

Address: _______________________________________

____

Notes: _______________________________________

____

____

Ear, Nose and Throat (ENT):

Name: _______________________________________

Phone: _______________________________________

Address: _______________________________________

____

Notes: _______________________________________

____

____

Audiologist:

Name: _______________________________________

Phone: _______________________________________

Address: _______________________________________

____

Notes: _______________________________________

____

____

Orthopedist:

Name: _______________________________________

Phone: _______________________________________

Address: _______________________________________

____

Notes: _______________________________________

____

____

Endocrinologist:

Name: _______________________________________

Phone: _______________________________________

Address: _______________________________________

____

Notes: _______________________________________

____

____

Gastroenterologist:

Name: _______________________________________

Phone: _______________________________________

Address: _______________________________________

____

Notes: _______________________________________

____

____

Allergist:

Name: ______________________________________

Phone: ______________________________________

Address: ____________________________________

____

Notes: ______________________________________

____

____

Nutritionist:

Name: ______________________________________

Phone: ______________________________________

Address: ____________________________________

____

Notes: ______________________________________

____

____

Cardiologist:

Name: ______________________________________

Phone: ______________________________________

Address: ____________________________________

____

Notes: ______________________________________

____

____

Dermatologist:

Name: ____

Phone: ____

Address: ____

____

Notes: ____

____

____

Physical Therapist:

Name: ____

Phone: ____

Address: ____

____

Notes: ____

____

____

Ocupational Therapist:

Name: ____

Phone: ____

Address: ____

____

Notes: ____

____

____

Sleep Clinic:

Name: ____

Phone: ____

Address: ____

____

Notes: ____

____

____

Pharmacy:

Name: ____

Phone: ____

Address: ____

____

Notes: ____

____

____

Hospital:

Name: ____

Phone: ____

Address: ____

____

Notes: ____

____

____

Other: _______________________________________

Name: ____

Phone: ____

Address: _______________________________________

____

Notes: ____

____

____

Other: _______________________________________

Name: ____

Phone: ____

Address: _______________________________________

____

Notes: ____

____

____

Other: _______________________________________

Name: ____

Phone: ____

Address: _______________________________________

____

Notes: ____

____

____

Baseline test

Baseline test must be done as soon as you get the Achondroplasia diagnosis to check for compression and apnea.

MRI of the brain and spine, with flexion and extension spinal flow study. (Page 36) (Page 39 Anesthesia)

-MRI of the brain and spine captures an image of the cranio cervical junction that may detect cervical cord compression.

-Flexion and extension allow the doctor to see the spine in the supine position and when it is bent up and down.

-Flow study allows evaluation of hydrocephalus and flow of cerebral spinal fluid around the brain, brainstem, and spinal cord.

-About Hydrocephalus (Page 43-44 / 58)

MRI Date: _______________________________________

Location: _______________________________________

Results: ____

____

Notes: ____

____

____

Polysomnography or sleep study. (Page 35-36-37) (Page 46-47)

-Monitors sleep stages and cycles.

-Identifies when and why sleep patterns are disrupted.

-Records brain waves, blood oxygen levels, heart rate, and breathing during sleep.

-Measures leg and arm movements.

-Be prepared to bring your pulse oximeter to the sleep study. Is good to know what is going on while your baby is doing sleep study.

-Before the sleep study ask the sleep clinics what procedures they do in case of emergencies like your kid having apneas and need oxygen. The clinics are not hospitals and may not carry these supplies.

-When the alarms sound, always check your child first. Never presume it is the machine having a problem. When the machine alarms, immediately check your child.

-Ask to include a ABG test (Page 35)

Sleep Study Date: _______________________________________

Location: ____

Results: ____

____

Notes: ____

____

____

Other important test:

BEAR test hearing test and follow-up every four to six months in first years of life. (Page 65-66)

Date: ____

Location: ____

Results: ____

____

Notes: ____

____

____

Spine X-Ray

    Date:____

    Location:_____________________________________

    Results: _____________________________________

    ____

    Note:____

    ____

    ____

Laryngoscope (Page 47)

    Date:____

    Location:_____________________________________

    Results _____________________________________

    ____

    Notes ______________________________________

    ____

    ____

Other:____

    Date:____

    Location:_____________________________________

    Results _____________________________________

    ____

    Notes ______________________________________

    ____

    ____

COMMON SURGERIES

Common surgeries and procedures your child may need in the first years.

Decompression surgery based on MRI results (Page 38-39-40)

Date:____

Location: ____

Results: ____

____

Notes: ____

____

____

Tonsillectomy and Adenoidectomy (Page 66)

Date: ____

Location: ____

Results: ____

____

Notes: ____

____

____

Ear tube placement (Page 66)

Date: ____

Location: ____

Results: ____

____

Notes: ____

____

____

MISCELLANEOUS

-Talk with a geneticist for approval on new items.
-Keep follow-up appointments with primary doctors and specialists.
-Do follow-up tests as ordered.
-Do not stress out with milestones because every child is different.
-Breastfeed your baby if you plan to do so and if medically okay.
-Give extra support to the head, neck, and back when breastfeeding, burping, and carrying.
-Learning to sew helps with altering clothing for age appropriateness.
-Have a balance; take care of your child; do not place them in a bubble.
-Enjoy your child.
-Do not let fear keep you apart from your child.
-Hug them, hold them, and enjoy them.
-This is a learning experience for everyone.
-Teach. Do not take comments personally.
-You are not alone.
-You have a wonderful community that is there for you and your family.
-Do not forget about yourself.
-Take time to process, rest, and keep going.
-Appointments, exams, new information, and the uknown are overwhelming.

You have got this!
Get ready because everything is going to be okay.

NOTES

NOTES

References

Children's Hospital of Philadelphia. (n.d.). Achondroplasia: Potential complications and risks. Retrieved from
https://www.chop.edu/conditions-diseases/achondroplasia

Chitty, L., Altman, D. (2002). Charts of fetal size: limb bones. Retrieved from International Journal of Obstetrics and Gynecology. Vol. 109, pp. 919-929.

Dubs, K. (2023). CPAP vs BiPAP Difference. How to know if you need a BiPAP Machine. Retrieved from www.cpap.com

Fact Sheet. (2017). Positioning and handling of babies with achondroplasia. Retrieved from
www.schn.health.nsw.gov.au/parents-macarer/factsheets/feedback-form

Geng, C. (2023). Medline Health News. Achondroplasia: Genetics and DNA Testing. Retrieved from
www.medicalnewstoday.com/articles/achondroplasiagenetics

Healthline. (2021). Epidural pros and cons. Retrieved from
https://www.healthline.com/health/pregnancy/epidural-prosand-cons

Johns Hopkins. (n.d.). Achondroplasia. Retrieved from
www.hopkinsmedicine.org/health/conditions-anddisease/achondroplasia

Johns Hopkins. (n.d.). Shunt Procedure. Retrieved from Neurology And Neurosurgery.
https://www.hopkinsmedicine.org/neurologyneurosurgery/centersclinics/cerebralfluid

Krucik, G., Ross, H. (2017). BAER (Brainstem Auditory Evoked Response) Test. Retrieved from https://www.healthline.com

Mayo Clinic. (n.d.). Atopic dermatitis (eczema). Retrieved from https://www.mayoclinic.org/diseasesconditions/atopicdermatitis

Mayo Clinic. (n.d.). Ear Tubes. Retrieved from www.mayoclinic.org/tests-procedures/eartubes

Mayo Clinic. (n.d.). Marfan syndrome. Retrieved from http://www.mayoclinic.org/diseases/conditions/marfansyndrome

Memorial Sloan Kettering Cancer Center. (n.d.). About Your Endoscopic Third Ventriculostomy (ETV) Surgery for Pediatric Patients. Retrieved from https://www.mskcc.org/cancer-care/patienteducation/about-your-etv-surgery

Medline Plus Medical Encyclopedia. (n.d.). HCG blood testqualitative. Retrieved from www.medlineplus.gov/ency/article/003509.htm

Morgan, K. (2021). What is Polysomnography (PSG)? Retrieved from https://www.webmd.com

MRI-Mayo Clinic. (n.d.). MRI. Retrieved from https://mayoclinic.org/tests-procedures/mri

Pereira, E., (2019. American Academy of Pediatrics. Achondroplasia. Retrieved from https://publications.aap.org/pediatrics

Ratini, M., MS. DO. (2022). Central Sleep Apnea. Retrieved from www.webmd.com/WebMDEditorialContributors

Raymondos, K., Seidel, T., Sander, B., Gerdes, A., Goetz, F., Helmstadter, V., Panning, B., Dieck, T. (2014). The intubation scoop (i-scoop)-a new type of laryngoscope for difficult and normal airways. Retrieved from https://pubmed.ncbi.nlm.nih.gov

Rekate, H. (2019). Pathogenesis of hydrocephalus in achondroplasia dwarfs: A review and presentation of a case followed for 22 years. Retrieved from National Library of Medicine. https://www.pubmed.ncbi.nlm.nih.gov

Sisk, E A., Heatley, D G., Borowski, B J., Leverson, G E., Pauli, R M. (1999). Obstructive sleep apnea in children with achondroplasia: surgical and anesthetic considerations. Retrieved from https://www.pubmed.ncbi.nlm.nih.gov

Spiegel, J., Hellman, M. (2015). Achondroplasia: Implications and Management Strategies in Anesthesia. Retrieved from https://www.anesthesiaexperts.com/uncategorized/achondro plasia-implications

Stanford Medicine Children's Health. (n.d.). Achondroplasia in Children. Retrieved from https://www.stanfordchildrens.org/en/topic/default/achondr o-plasia

Sydney Children's Hospital Network. (n.d.). Retrieved from https://www.schn.health.nsw.gov.au.factsheets/achondroplas i-a-position

Vaughn, D. (2023). Foramen-Magnum. Retrieved from https://www.Britannica.com/2023/science/foramen-magnum

9 798337 696720